WHEELING AROUND THE BLUEGRASS

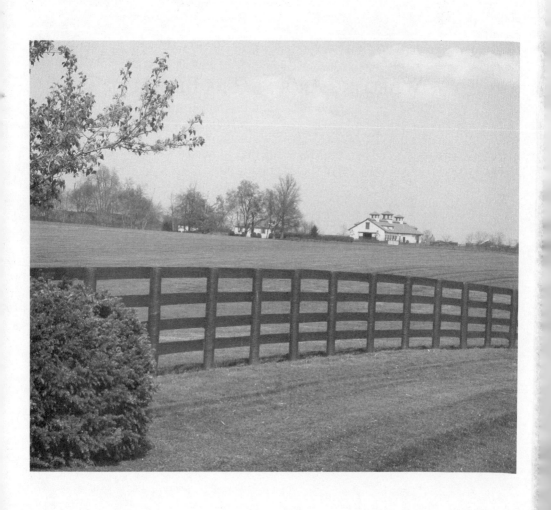

Joe Ward

Wheeling Around The Bluegrass

BUTLER BOOKS

To the Bluegrass Cycling Club, a good group of people to get a person rolling.

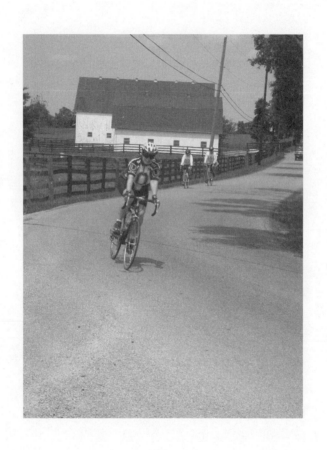

Table of Contents

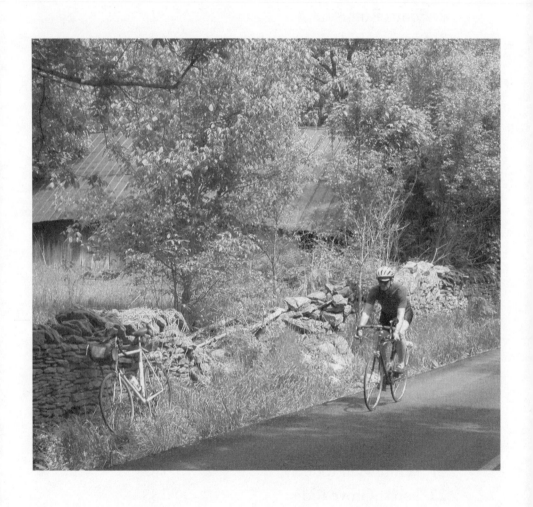

INTRODUCTION

The first thing most people think of when you mention The Bluegrass as a region is horses. And understandably so. The ground in The Bluegrass is underlain with limestone, which dissolves and imparts calcium phosphate and calcium magnesium carbonate into the soil and water. It's great for livestock of all kinds, and especially for horses, because it promotes strong but light bones and tendons. So there is a greater concentration of horse farms in The Bluegrass than in any other part of the world.

In the inner Bluegrass, around Lexington, and mostly near Keeneland race course just west of Lexington, the horse farms are unbelievable. They actually look a little unreal, green, green grass viewed across carefully restored 19th century stone fences, or plank fences painted white or black that cost $20,000 a mile, carefully husbanded grounds, and incredible barns painted in pastel colors, their rooflines bristling with cupolas.

Here and there there's an old mansion peeking through the trees, white columns gleaming, chimneys soaring, a groomed drive winding up from a signature gate. It's a feast for the eyes to be sure, and most of it very accessible by bicycle. People who settled in The Bluegrass grew prosperous early, and they built lots of roads to get from farm to market, from home to church and from village to village. Even after the coming of the big highways later, those old roads have been preserved and paved, and the really thick, fast traffic mostly bypasses their interconnected meanderings. In short, it's a cyclist's dream. Roads to ride in all sorts of combinations and lengths. Sights to see at every turn. Here and there a country grocery for a rest and a cold drink, and maybe a sandwich.

But the horses are by no means all of it. The Bluegrass covers a large area. You can ride past goat farms in Mercer County, and see cattle grazing on the hillsides as you ride the ridge tops of Robertson County. Knobs poke up all around you as you pedal through the Red Lick Valley in Estill County, and there are ancient farmsteads to view along the North Rolling Fork of the Salt River in northern Casey County.

There are well-paved, interconnected back roads throughout, to give you a long ride or short, your choice. There are hills enough to keep the terrain from being boring, but few hills high and steep enough to make you not want to go there.

And everywhere there is history. This is the motherland for the U.S. west of the Alleghenies. Here Americans finally broke out of the eastern seaboard, and began the westward march that made the U.S. a great country. Later, it was a crossroads in the sad struggle that kept the country together. So you can't go anywhere in The Bluegrass without crossing the trail of Daniel Boone, or John Hunt Morgan.

Boone, in particular, was all over this country, starting in 1769 when he arrived with a party of hunters and then stayed here alone while they went back to North Carolina for supplies. He checked the whole country out, from the Falls of the Ohio to the Blue Licks, to the headwaters of the Salt River. He noted where the cane grew tall because he knew the fertile land would be there.

I gather from reading up on him for this book that he also used the canebrakes for cover a lot, as did the Indians he was carefully trying to avoid. Whenever there was a scrape of any kind, everybody, Indians and whites, would jump into the canebrakes, and usually get away. Apparently cane grew like corn in a field, only sometimes it was 30 feet high. And not even a Shawnee warrior wanted to go into the canebrakes after someone hiding with a gun, a knife, and a hatchet. It was hard to find such a person, and that was the good news. I think cane should be the state plant.

But I'm wandering here. My goal with this book is to get you to ride through the Bluegrass and taste it for yourself. If you live around here, I hope you'll give the countryside a look from the saddle of a bicycle. You get a really enjoyable view. If you live somewhere else, I hope you'll come here on vacation - maybe take a week or so and do as many of these rides as you can. You'll realize much more of the benefit to be had from visiting here than if you stick to your car.

Besides local people and visitors, I also aimed this book at both beginners and experienced cyclists. I've made a sincere effort here to be all things to all people. By beginners, I mean people who maybe ride bicycles around the block now and then, and mean to get out and get some real exercise, but haven't somehow managed to do that. It's a group that I need to buy this book, because there are so many of you. So I scrutinized favorite rides from early in my cycling career—which started in The Bluegrass almost 30 years ago—and rides suggested to me by members of the Lexington-based Bluegrass Cycling Club, for short pieces that could be pulled out to stand alone as exquisite nuggets. I whittled one ride out of Keeneland down to just over 6 miles, in a particularly heroic effort. But mostly the short rides are between 10 and 15 miles. Here's a list of them, with page numbers where they can be found:

Short Keeneland Ride. 6 miles. Page 20
Short Old Whiskey Trail Ride. 11 miles. Page 48
Short Jot 'Em Down Ride. 10 miles. Page 58
Short Paris-Beth-Paris. 15 miles. Page 68
Short Switzer Bridge Ride.12 miles (but there could be some hills.)
    Page 82
Short Trail of the Lonesome Pine. 12 miles. Page 108
Short Cane Ridge Ride. 14 miles. Page 114
Short Perryville Battlefield Ride. 13 miles. Page 170
High Bridge Ride. 15 miles. Page 198

While I kept that one eye on the huge numbers of beginning cyclists, I also knew that, in general, it will be easier to sell this book to experienced cyclists. They're already looking for the very thing this book has—a few good rides with a little information about what there is to look at along the way, and where to stop for a few minutes to get an Ale-8-One. (For you non-Bluegrass people, that's a little insider reference to a ginger-flavored soft drink bottled in Winchester, Ky., and widely available in The Bluegrass, but hardly anywhere else. My wife, Suzanne, claims it aids digestion.)

Unlike beginners, experienced cyclists tend to want to get out and ride all day, and maybe do that several days in a row. So I put in some longer rides for them. And I supplied some connector routes so riders can string together the main rides, and actually ride for days. By using the connectors, a rider could start at Owingsville, on the eastern edge of The Bluegrass, ride by a meandering path down to West Irvine, in the southeast, and pedal west through Berea, Harrodsburg and Perryville to Penn's Store, near Gravel

Switch, on the southwest edge of The Bluegrass. He could then head up through Cornishville and Lawrenceburg, Versailles, Switzer and Paris, and up to Mt. Olivet on the northern edge of The Bluegrass. The links are described in detail starting at page 219.

What you're supposed to do with this book is sit down and read the narrative while looking at the map and the route sheet. When you're thinking about a ride, photocopy the map and the route sheet, and look at them as you read. Check out all of the turns. See where the stores are. Check the mileage. Then save the photocopies to clip on your handlebars for easy reference as you ride along.

TIPS

Here's how to make a handle bar, or stem, clip to hold your maps. Go to an office supply place and get a binder clamp such as you see in the illustration, and some of those nylon ties that have teeth to hold on snugly once they've been pulled into place. Strap one of the wire bales of the clip to the bicycle stem with one of the ties, so that the clip opens back toward the saddle. Pull the tie tight, and trim off the loose end. Wrap a piece of plastic tape around the bale and the tie for a neat appearance. Use the other bale to pry the clip open, insert your map or route sheet, and you're in business. The maps have been drawn and the route sheets printed to be of a good size for the stem clip— not so big they'll flop around a lot, but big enough 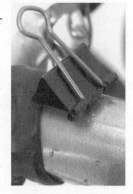 that you can glance at them while you're riding. Be careful, though. Detailed study should be reserved for stops.

About those horse farms. They are open to visitors in many cases, but they are working farms and they like to know when you're coming. You should call ahead and make an appointment. If you want to visit several farms and aren't sure of your riding pace or that of your group, it might be hard to design a schedule that will work well. So, sad to say, while cycling is certainly the best way to see most of the horse country, it may not be the best way to visit farms. In the ride narratives I mention specific farms about which I knew or could find interesting tidbits of information. But I haven't tried to include a comprehensive listing of all the farms these rides go past. There are about 450 horse farms in the area.

While some of the farms are quite venerable and famous, some of those most heavily involved in what's going on in the horse world now are quite new. Farms actually change hands fairly often. Attitudes toward visitors are subject to change as well, with seasons or with events. The Lexington Convention and Visitors Bureau keeps track of all this, and its web site—www.visitlex.com—is the best place to find up-to-date information. It is quite user-friendly and comprehensive.

A good way to get a quick, broad look at the horse farm culture is to visit the **Kentucky Horse Park,** which is on Ironworks Pike, just east of I-75, about four miles north of Lexington. It includes a working farm that has many breeds of horses, and a wonderful museum that traces man's relationship with the equine race from the beginnings of time to the present. The park also plays host to special exhibits from time to time, each of them a once-in-a-lifetime opportunity. I didn't put the horse park on any of the rides in this book because Ironworks Pike has become quite busy right near the park, and riding there is not as much fun as it used to be.

But there is a campground at the park that would offer a fairly central location to stay for camping cyclists looking over these rides. And any visitor would find it well worth the time to drive to the park and look it over. You probably shouldn't expect to spend too much time riding the day you go to the park. There's a lot to see there.

Road bikes, the kind with the skinny tires and saddles, and drop-type handlebars are probably best for the rides in this book. Mountain bikes would be okay for some of the shorter ones, but the rolling resistance from their thick and heavy tires would prove wearing on anything over 15 or 16 miles. A road bike puts your body in an efficient position for pedaling many miles with less fatigue. "You're like a runner," Dr. Grace Donnelly, my cycling mentor in the Bluegrass club years ago, used to say. You're leaning forward in an attitude of motion rather than one of sitting. The posture permits you to distribute your weight evenly between the pedals, handlebar and saddle

—which is the secret of comfortable riding on those skinny saddles. If you're riding properly, a wide saddle will actually chafe the insides of your thighs, which can make you quite uncomfortable over several hours time.

My friend Tom Armstrong, a leading area proponent of recumbent bicycles—the kind you sort of lie back in and pedal with your legs up in the air—would hold me remiss if I didn't say you probably could do any of these rides on a recumbent, too. I have limited experience with recumbents myself, but judging by the pace and distance at which I've seen Tom and others ride them with no apparent ill effect, I guess I have to say you probably could.

I recommend **Effective Cycling** methods for riding in general. By that I mean the approach to cycling transportation outlined in the book *Effective Cycling* by John Forester—available in a bookstore near you. The basic idea is to ride by essentially the same rules of the road as you would when driving a car. One difference is that, on a bicycle, you treat each lane as if it were two. When riding on the right side of a four-lane road, for example, if you wanted to turn left, you would move into the left lane in a series of steps. Check for traffic from behind and move from the right side of the right lane to the left side of the right lane. Check again and move to the right side of the left lane, then make your turn and move over to the right side of the right lane on the new road.

Anybody on a bicycle should wear a **helmet** approved by the Consumer Products Safety Commission. It's far enough from where you're sitting to the pavement to crack your skull if you should land on it. There were two cycling helmets available when I started cycling—a Bell and an MSR. Now there are hundreds, in bewildering assortment, from a few dollars to totally ridiculous. The safety certification is the main thing to look for.

Next after a helmet you need **gloves** with padded leather palms. They absorb some of the shock from hours on the handlebar, and also protect the palms of your hands from gravel in the event of a crash. They're readily available in bike shops from about $10 up. You'll need **cycling shoes**, too, something with a stiff sole that will keep the pedal from cutting off the circulation in the sole of your foot. Many bicycles now come with various types of clipless pedals. If you have a set of those, you'll need to get shoes that match the pedals. For old-fashioned toe clips, the type of shoes now sold as "SPD compatible" will work. Just don't bother to install the cleats.

Unless you own a van or a pickup, you will need some sort of **bike rack** for your car to get your bike or bikes to the starting places of these rides. Such racks also are readily available, at bike shops and discount stores, in models that go on the back of the car, on top, or on a trailer hitch. You can get a usable rack from about $40 to about $300. I personally also like a carrier on the bike, a rigid one that goes behind the saddle over the back wheel, for rides like these. You never know when you're going to want to buy something at some little store on the way. They cost $25 to $50 at bike shops, and are easy to bolt on.

You will need a **spare inner tube**, and a **tire patch kit**, and the knowledge to use both. Those skinny tires cut down on the rolling resistance very well, but they are thin and easier to puncture than other tires. When you look down and notice that you're riding through a patch of shattered glass where some thoughtful soul has thrown a bottle down, you should stop, in fact, and clear both of your tires with your leather palm. Otherwise, a small piece of glass can become imbedded and work its way through the tire with the revolutions of the wheel. You'll need a **tire pump** that you can mount on the frame of your bicycle. Make sure it fits the type of valve you have on your tires. Pumps start at about $20 at bike shops. Your tire patch kit should include tire levers for removing the tire from the wheel rim. It's a good idea to have a **screw driver and hex wrenches,** as well, and maybe a small adjustable wrench along for other things that might go wrong. Small tool bags that fit under the saddle are available to keep it all organized.

A **cyclometer** of some sort is also a great help on rides like these. While no two cyclometers ever read the same after about a mile and a half of travel, they can give you an idea if you are totally off course. I give mileage figures on the route sheets to the tenth of a mile, but those are really only ball-park figures. If a particular corner doesn't come up right on schedule, you should not worry immediately. If you go a couple of miles without seeing something you are supposed to be seeing, it's time to stop and try to figure out where you are. Cyclometers are available from about $15 and up. Some have heart rate monitors, for serious training, and some even have altimeters, if you want to really document your suffering.

Speaking of which, be sure also to take along a **water bottle**, especially for a long ride. Dehydration can be dangerous. Bottles with cages to be bolted on the bike frame are readily available, as are water packs that you wear on your back with a hose to your mouth. Those are mostly used for very long rides, such as "centuries," which are 100 miles long. You usually can refill your water bottle at a country store or service station. In a pinch, experienced cyclists often look around the exterior foundations of country churches for working spigots. The church is not likely to miss a bottle or so of water, but you have to judge whether such water is safe. Take along something to snack on too. Drink before you're thirsty. Eat before you're hungry.

Bike shops in the bluegrass seem to be mostly in Lexington, though I found one business in Richmond that offers bicycles and parts: Outback Sports, 2780 Tates Creek Rd., 727-819-8708. And there is one in Danville: Danville Bike & Fitness, 417 W. Main Street, 859-238-7669.

These are the Lexington shops:
Dodds Cyclery & Fitness, 1985 Harrodsburg Rd. Phone: (859) 277-6013
Pedal Power Bike Shop, 401 S. Upper St. Phone: (859) 255-6408
Scheller's Fitness & Cycling, 212 Woodland Ave. Phone: (859) 233-1764
Tenth Gear Bicycle Shop, 521 Southland Dr. Phone: (859) 278-1053
Vicious Cycle, 3090 Todds Rd. Suite 306. Phone: (859) 263-7300

The Bluegrass has been a destination for cyclists since bicycles were invented. Karl Kron cycled down from Cincinnati, through Georgetown and Lexington, to Shakertown and Perryville on his way to Mammoth Cave on a high-wheel bicycle in 1882. Kron, a New Yorker and graduate of Yale whose real name was Lyman Hotchkiss Bagg, wrote about his trip in an 1887 book called *Ten Thousand Miles on a Bicycle*. He said this:

"The foliage of the trees—which do not often form thickly interlacing 'woods,' but stand out alone in their individual majesty, as if some magnificent landscape-gardiner had designedly stationed them there to form the symmetrical landmarks and ornaments of an immense park— was brilliantly verdant; and the tall grass, which gives its peculiar name to that section of the state, shone, if I may say so, with the bluest green imaginable."

Among other things, Kron said he stopped in Lexington to visit with the president of the local cycling club, and tried to stop at "the Shaker Settlement" for the night. But he said he got to Shakertown after dark and there wasn't a single light in the "big white houses" of the village. He'd been told one of the houses was "accustomed to entertaining strangers," but he couldn't be sure which it was, so he lost his nerve and went on to Harrodsburg. There he did manage to roust an innkeeper, but that wasn't easy, either.

In 1896, when the **League of American Wheelmen** was holding its annual "meet" in Louisville—an event that drew 30,000 people, by *The Courier-Journal*'s estimate—the Courier ran a long article to let visitors know where to find good riding in the state. "A trip to Lexington and the Bluegrass region, 'God's Country,' will be an experience well worth devoting two or three days to," it said. "No ride awheel will compare to it."

I formed the same opinion in 1975, when—following the advice of riders in the Bluegrass Wheelmen club—I bought a bike that fit me and began doing rides farther than around the block. The club has since been renamed the Bluegrass Cycling Club, but it's still there. And a number of its members helped me put together this collection of rides for you. They host the Horsey Hundred invitational ride every year just before Memorial Day and draw hundreds of riders to The Bluegrass from all over the country, and from foreign countries. You can learn more about it at the ride's website: http://www.bgcycling.org/horsey/

While you're at it, you might check out the Kentucky Rails to Trails Council's web page at www.KyRailTrail.org. They are trying to convert an old railroad bed that runs east from Lexington to the Ashland area—right through a wonderful stretch of the country this book is about—into a trail for cycling and other activities.

Meanwhile, it's your turn to head out for some wheeling in The Bluegrass. Enjoy.

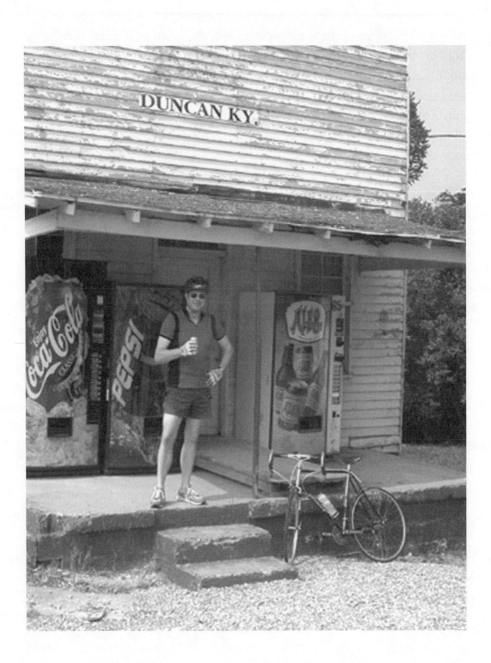

25 Rides
(and a bonus Tour de France)

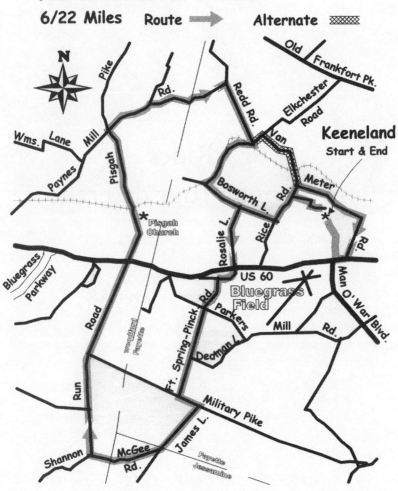

Keeneland Ride

6/22 Miles   Route ➡   Alternate ▨▨▨

N

Pike
Rd.
Redd Rd.
Old
Frankfort Pk.
Elkchester
Road

Van

Keeneland
Start & End

Wms. Lane
Mill
Paynes
Pisgah

Bosworth L.
Rd.
Meter

Rice

* Pisgah
Church

Rosalie L.

Bluegrass
Parkway

US 60

Man O' War Blvd.

**Bluegrass
Field**

Road
woodford
Fayette

Ft. Spring-Pinck. Rd.
Parkers
Mill
Rd.

Dedman L.

Run

Military Pike

Shannon
McGee
Rd.
James L.
Fayette
Jessamine

1
Keeneland Ride

Six or 22 miles. Some hills. Crosses one busy road. Start in the barn parking lot at Keeneland, off Versailles Road, 1.5 miles west of Lexington. Enter opposite Man O' War Boulevard.

The Bluegrass region is the heart of Kentucky, and **Keeneland,** the race track, is the heart of the Bluegrass. It's a very good place to find fast horses, beautiful women, and good whiskey, especially during the spring and fall racing meetings, in April and October.

But it's a good place to start a bicycle ride any time of year, and a bit less crowded the other 10 months. You can find very expensive horses running on the training track about any time. And the track kitchen, where you can find owners, trainers, and jockeys, not to mention grooms and hot walkers, eating a country breakfast any time of year, is open to the general public.

You have to get there fairly early, though. It's open from 6 to 11 a.m. most of the year, with a bit of an extension to cover lunch during racing meetings and sales. The food is good, varied and plentiful, the price is right, and the atmosphere very appealing—especially in early summer when the grass is really blue.

And That's Just the Start

There's really no better taste of the Bluegrass horse farm country than right around Keeneland. Some of the really huge spreads, with barns that cost several times the price of most peoples' houses, are a bit farther

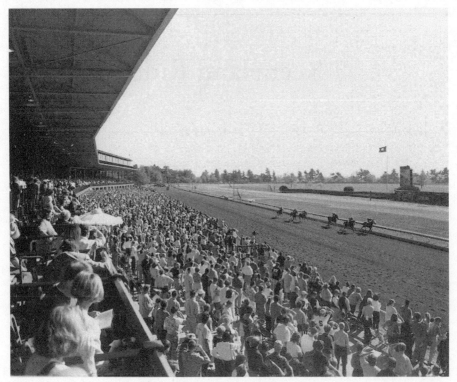

The stands at Keeneland racecourse.

Keeneland Photo

out, and we'll pass some of them in later rides.

But the improbable, park-like flavor of horse country is readily available right here. You ride along un-crowded, well-paved roads, past plank fences and old stone walls, and beautiful mares with prancing foals in every direction. My friend and former colleague, **Doug Perry** wrote of a farm not far from the track, that he would have been "only mildly surprised to see a unicorn go bounding by."

Sometimes you actually do wonder if it can be real, or is maybe some huge theme park. It's real. So Keeneland is a fitting place to start this Bluegrass book, with the shortest ride it has to offer. It will take you about six miles—depending on how much you wander around the parking lot— to cycle around some of the area closest to the track.

It's the heart of a 22-mile ride shown to me by my friend, **Bill Fortune**, a **University of Kentucky** law professor, and noted cyclist with the Bluegrass club.

Million-dollar Babies

First, there's Keeneland, itself. It is perhaps best known for its races, which offer millions of dollars in purses each summer and fall, and attract thousands of patrons to a laid-back, open racing experience that provides the public with easy access to paddock and barns—which few tracks permit.

But, in addition to its race meetings, Keeneland also sells a lot of high-priced horseflesh at six sales a year. Hundreds of millions of dollars worth. I was occasionally pressed into service to cover the sales in my days as a Courier-Journal reporter, when a horse-beat colleague couldn't make it. I noticed that the regular racing reporters there didn't seem to pay much attention until the bidding got up to about $1 million.

They didn't actually get agitated, and start looking around for the sheiks and high-rolling Irish until it got to $3 million or $4 million. It's an exciting thing to watch.

The Goods on Seabiscuit

What is less well known is that Keeneland has an incredible racing library where writers of all types—from everywhere—come when they really want to know about horses and speed. It contains the donated personal libraries of many prominent horse people of the past, all of the editions of such publications as the Daily Racing Form, and a treasury of other documents.

Laura Hillenbrand, who wrote *Seabiscuit: An American Legend* — which became a best-selling book and a great movie—did a lot of research at Keeneland. She noted that the great moments of horse racing—the thundering last minutes in the stretch at the Kentucky Derby, for example—pass very quickly. Then they exist only in memory and in history, she said, and at Keeneland's library.

Keeneland was started in 1935 by a group of horsemen. It plows all of its profits back into the track with improvements or larger purses, or gives them to charity.

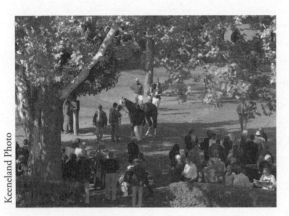

Keeneland Photo

The Paddock at Keeneland.

Man O' War Entrance.

The best way to start a ride from Keeneland is to head into the big parking lot by the barns by taking a right turn off U.S. 60—Versailles Road—across from Man O' War Boulevard about a mile and a half west of **Lexington's** New Circle Road. Go in there and find a place to park. Parking is free. It shouldn't be hard to find a place, especially if there's no racing meet on—though you get the best flavor of the place if it is.

Wander around and find the track kitchen. If you're doing this right, you'll be early enough to have some eggs and bacon, or biscuits and gravy, or cereal with fruit. Or, if you're really early, or doing the short route, you could eat after you get back.

Trainers are often working horses on the training track at 6 a.m., track kitchen assistant manager **Josie Clark** told me. "It's sort of a ritual for people to come out and eat and go watch them," she said.

Head for Rice Road

Once you're on your bicycle, you can sort of use the track water tower, visible from about anywhere on the 907-acre property, to guide you. Go past the blacksmith shop and turn left at the water tower.

Head out the gate and turn left on Rice Road. The training track is down along Rice Road. Take a right off Rice onto Bosworth Lane. If you're on the longer ride, take a left on Rosalie Lane, up the hill. More about that direction later.

You short-ride people just stay straight on Bosworth Lane until you cross the tracks and meet Elkchester Road. See that marvelous house on the right with all of the turrets and garrets and the porch all around. Bill Fortune said it belongs to a veterinarian with a practice over in Versailles, who apparently is just a flamboyant person.

You take Elkchester up past Redd Road, which will come in on the left, to a right turn on Van Meter Road, KY 1969. As you approach the intersection of Van Meter and Rice roads, you'll be passing **Drumkenny Farm** on your right. It's a relative newcomer to the area, in operation since 1996.

Buy Low, Sell High

The name Drumkenny is a combination of the home towns in Ireland and Scotland of **Patrick and Lynne Costello**, who own and operate the farm. They board and breed mares. They also work with a group of investors called "**The Lads,**" who buy weanlings and try to sell them as yearlings at a profit. They bought the filly **Gold Fever** for $70,000 and sold her for $600,000. They bought **Chris S**. for $100,000, and sold him for $900,000. You see how this business works.

On down Van Meter, on the left, you have **Fares Farm**. There are 900 acres there. They board and train horses, and prepare them for sale. It will cost you $22 a day to have your weanling, broodmare or yearling stay there. But if you have a foal that hasn't been weaned with your mare, that's free. Sales prep is $30 a day, and training to race is $35 a day.

On down the road, Van Meter takes a bend, and you find yourself riding along the white plank fences and white barns with Devil Red trim of Calumet Farm, the most storied horse farm in the Bluegrass. They've bred a record nine Kentucky Derby winners there, including the Triple Crown winners **Whirlaway** and **Citation**. That's how people really keep score in the horse business.

The Glorious 1940s

Calumet's real glory was in the 1940s, when **Warren Wright Sr.** ran the place. His father, **William Monroe Wright**, was the founder of the **Calumet Baking Powder Co.**, which his son sold for $40 million. The son put a lot of the money into good thoroughbreds.

He bought a share of a stallion named **Blenheim II**, who became the sire of Whirlaway. Whirlaway won the Triple Crown in 1941. Wright bought **Bull Lea** at the Saratoga yearling sale for $14,000, and he fathered Citation, generally considered second only to **Man O' War** among the great horses of the 20th century. He won the Triple Crown in 1947.

Calumet hasn't had a decade like that since, actually, and though it has bred and owned more Derby winners than any other farm, it found itself on the auction block facing debts of more than $100 million in 1992. Along came **Henryk de Kwaitkowski**, a native of Poland with a fairly interesting history himself, to buy the farm at auction for $17 million.

Flying Spitfires with the Royal Air Force

According to the farm's official biography, Kwaitkowski was born in Warsaw, and shipped off to a work camp in Siberia when the Russians invaded Poland in 1939, when he was 15. A couple of years later he escaped through Iran and made it to a Canadian ship, which was torpedoed en route to England. He was one of the few survivors.

He made it to England and lied about his age to join two of his six brothers in the RAF, flying spitfires. Eventually, he studied at Cambridge and in Canada, became an aeronautical engineer, and got rich in the airplane business.

The entire Bluegrass breathed a sigh of relief when he bought Calumet, name and all, and announced that its 30 miles of white fences would remain white as long as he lived. That turned out to be until March of 2003, when he died at 79. The farm was in trust as this book was written.

The Rest of the Story

Once past Calumet, you can take a right at U.S. 60 - the shoulder's nice to ride on there, down to Man O' War Boulevard, for another right back into Keeneland's parking lot.

For those who are up for a longer ride, though, this narrative will now return to the corner of Bosworth Lane and Rosalie Lane, where you will turn left, up the hill. Rosalie takes you down to U.S. 60, which can be tricky to cross at that point, depending on the time of day. There is room to stop out in the middle of the four lanes, so you can take them in two darts if you have to—as riders in the Bluegrass Cycling Club's Horsey Hundred invitational ride often do each May.

Once across, you find yourself on Old Versailles Road, in the community of **Fort Spring**. You can tell it's an old place, especially the stone building on your right just as you take a left on Fort Spring-Pinckard Road. There was a mill, a store, and some taverns here in the early 1800s. The place was called Slickaway in those days. Its post office took the name Fort Springs in 1886, and closed in 1903.

BCC Stomping Grounds

The Bluegrass Cycling Club, which was the Bluegrass Wheelmen in my day, rides the roads in here a lot. In fact, you're likely to see the road markings from the Horsey anywhere along here.

I've always enjoyed what seems like an abrupt change from hustling, bustling civilization to the boondocks when you duck down Fort Springs Road. Actually, it's easy to miss, so start watching for it as soon as you get across U.S. 60

It takes you across Parkers Mill and Dedman Lane, both frequently-used cycling roads, to a leftward jog on Military Pike, and a right turn on James Lane. That goes up to McGee Road. (The sign there says McGee Road II, for some reason.) Turn to the right there and pedal over to Shannon Run Road.

You'll see signs for **Garrett's Orchard**, which has been a frequent ride destination and is a good place to find fruit and vegetables at various times of the year. Shannon Run takes you back across U.S. 60, only with a traffic light this time. You may have to wait for a motor vehicle to trip it for you, though.

The Castle

Once you're across, look up to the right for a good view of Woodford County's castle, a sort of mysterious landmark that has attracted attention from passersby since the early 1970s. I was in *The Courier-Journal's* Bluegrass

Bureau in those days, and I remember we tried mightily to get a story on the place, without much success.

It was built by a developer named **Rex Martin**, who had traveled with his wife, **Caroline**, in Europe and become enamored with castles. When we'd call, he'd always beg off, saying the place wasn't really anything like it was going to be, and that it would make a much better story later.

A story went around that Caroline wanted her existing house on a garden tour, but it didn't measure up. So Martin promised to build her a place that nobody could take off the garden tour.

Unfortunately, the couple divorced in 1975, and the castle was never finished. News stories over the years say Martin moved to Florida and put the place up for sale, but never has shown much interest in actually making a deal on it. The asking price is said to be just under $1 million. Martin died as this book was being written.

Another story went around that people in the entourage of **Queen Elizabeth II** of England—who sometimes visits her horses at nearby **Lane's End Farm**—don't think the castle looks much like a real one. The person reportedly said it would not be a surprise to see **Donald Duck** peeking over the wall.

Old Pisgah

You've been on Pisgah Pike since crossing U.S. 60, named for the **Pisgah Presbyterian Church**, which you will soon come to. It's sort of a revered landmark in the area. The congregation was organized in 1784, and this stone church building put up in 1812. It was extensively renovated in a Gothic style in 1868. Seven soldiers from the Revolutionary War are buried in the cemetery by the church door.

The churchyard also has the grave of **A.B. "Happy" Chandler,** from nearby Versailles, who was Kentucky governor twice and U.S. senator once.

There's a bit of a rough railroad crossing just past the church. Be careful. The place on the left is the home of **Ben Chandler**, grandson of Happy. As this book was being written, Ben Chandler was a candidate for governor himself. So, as you read this, he may be running the state. Or not.

Trotters

On the right along there is **Brittany Farm**, which breeds Standardbred, trotting, horses. Among its products are **Self Possessed**, the fastest winner ever of the **Hambletonian**, the breed's premiere race. The Hambletonian has been around since 1926, and William M. Wright, of Calumet was one of its founders. It has been run at **Meadowlands**, in New Jersey, since 1981.

Brittany Farms also bred **Continentalvictory**, another Hambletonian winner, and the fastest three-year-old trotting filly in history.

There is a lot of great country all along here - turn right on Paynes Mill Road and just take in the fences and the barns and the houses, and the green, green pastures. Turn right on Redd Road, and then cut right again on Elkchester, to go down past the previously-mentioned home of the Versailles vet, with all of its turrets and garrets.

Take Bosworth back to Rice, but don't turn in to Keeneland. Go on by to pick up Van Meter, and the ride past historic Calumet. Then take the short piece of U.S. 60's shoulder and you're back at Keeneland.

Welcome to wheeling in The Bluegrass.

Route Sheet

0.0	Left on Rice Road out the back gate of Keeneland
0.1	Right on Bosworth Lane
0.8	Left on Rosalie Road, up the hill
1.7	Straight across Versailles Road to Old Versailles Road Be careful.
2.0	Left on Fort Springs-Pinckard Road
2.7	Cross Parkers Mill Road. Stay straight.
4.2	Left on Military Pike
4.5	Right on James Lane
5.9	Right on McGee Road II
6.9	Right on Shannon Run Road
8.5	Pass Military Pike on the right.
10.1	Cross U.S. 60 with the light. Be careful. Notice castle up on the right.
10.8	Pisgah Church
12.6	Right on Paynes Mill Road
13.4	Turning climb out of creek
14.3	Right turn on Redd Road
15.3	Right on Elkchester Road
15.8	Vet's house
16.2	Follow Elkchester to right at tracks.
16.4	Left on Bosworth Lane
17.1	Pass Rosalie.
17.8	Left on Rice Road. Go on past the gate to Keeneland.
19.5	Right on Van Meter Road
20.6	Calumet Farm is on the left
21.3	Right on the shoulder of U.S. 60
21.5	Right on Man O' War Blvd., into Keeneland
21.7	Left into parking lot

Keeneland Short Ride

0.0	Left on Rice Road out of the Keeneland Gate
0.1	Right on Bosworth Lane
1.5	Right on Elkchester Road, after tracks
2.5	Right on Van Meter Road (KY 1969)
5.9	Right on U.S. 60 shoulder
6.1	Right on Man O' War, back into Keeneland

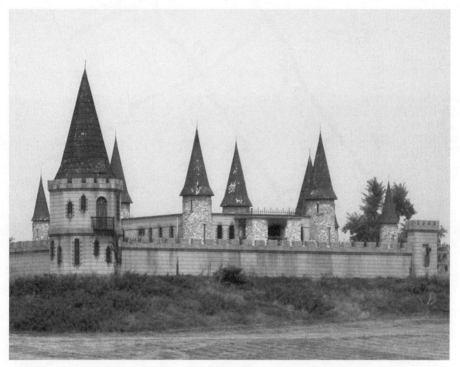

The late Rex Martin's castle near Keeneland.

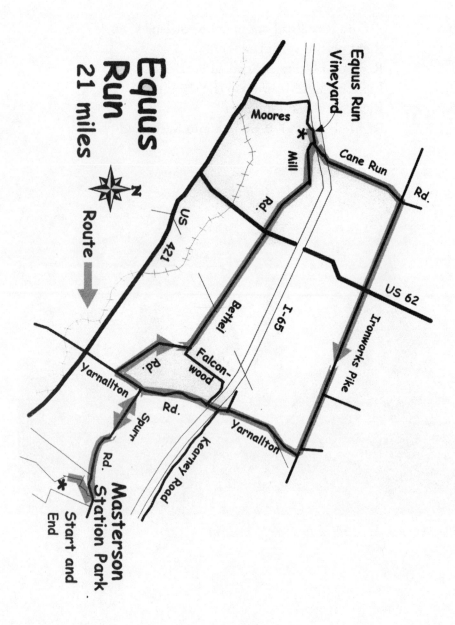

Equus
Run
21 miles

N

Route →

Equus Run
Vineyard

Moores

Cane Run

Mill

Rd.

Rd.

US 62

US 421

Bethel

I-65

Ironworks Pike

Falcon-
wood

Rd.

Yarnallton

Spurr

Rd.

Yarnallton

Kearney Road

Rd.

Masterson
Station Park

Start and
End

2

Equus Run Ride

Twenty-one miles. Few Hills. Moderate Traffic. Start at the soccer complex parking lot in Masterson Station Park, a bit over two miles northwest of Lexington's New Circle Road on U.S. 421.

This is another nice Inner-Bluegrass ride done frequently by the Bluegrass Club and outlined for me by Bill Fortune. You might want to take along a few sandwiches or some bread, sausage and cheese, because the vineyard for which the ride is named offers prime picnic sites in the grass under the trees along a meandering stream. You can also taste the wine.

The ride starts out at Masterson Station Park, a large area of playing fields given to Lexington by the federal government, after it converted an old narcotics hospital on part of the property of a federal prison in the early 1970s. The whole area is still often referred to as "Narco."

It's always easy to find a place to park by the soccer complex, which is reached by a park road from the park entrance on Leestown Road, which is U.S. 421. From there you start riding on the park road on to Shamrock Road, still in the park, and take that past the stables. You can sign up for horse riding lessons there, incidentally, if you get a hankering for a different kind of saddle.

Shamrock Road reaches Spurr Road, and you turn left.

Rehabilitating Men and Horses

As you turn left on Spurr, you get a glimpse on your right of

33

Blackburn Correctional Complex, a 390-bed minimum security prison, where inmates work with retired Thoroughbreds, among other things.

The state set aside 100 prime Bluegrass acres, of Blackburn's 360, for a program operated by the **Thoroughbred Retirement Foundation**, which also has similar programs at correctional facilities in other horse states.

Horses that have raced and are in danger of ending up in a glue factory, or meeting some similarly inappropriate fate, can be sent to the program, where they will be cared for in their old age. Men who qualify for the program—which is to say, 50 to 60 from Blackburn's population—work with the horses, learning skills that may get them jobs when their prison time is up.

In the process, they undergo healing as well, learning how to accept responsibility and getting a boost in their feeling of self-worth.

The Old Narcotics Farm

And on your left, as you pedal along, you'll see the buildings of the old federal narcotics hospital, which once produced a lot for its own support on much of the farmland in this area.

It became a federal prison in 1974, and was converted to a federal medical center in 1991. It accepts patients from other institutions in the federal prison system, many of whom require specialized care.

In its prison days, a few famous inmates rotated through. One was **Otto Kerner**, a former Illinois governor and head of an important federal advisory commission on civil disorder. He was convicted in the early 1970s of bribery, perjury and a few other things in connection with a race track stock deal.

Another was **Lynette "Squeaky" Fromme**, a **Charles Manson** disciple who tried to kill U.S. President **Gerald Ford** in 1975.

Notice the warden's house, up on the hill to your left. Nice digs. That's the medical center behind it.

There are Horse Farms, Too

On Spurr Road across from the federal hospital is **Crestwood Farm**,

34

owned by **Pope McLean,** who operates it with three grown children. Crestwood's top stud is **Storm Boot,** a son of **Storm Cat,** who was about the hottest stallion around as this was being written.

The success of Storm Boot's progeny at race tracks had enabled the McLeans to raise his stud fee from $1,000 to $15,000 in a few steps. The writer of a 2002 profile of the McLeans in **The Blood Horse** magazine said that progression may have been a first.

The Blood Horse quoted Pope McLean saying that if more people could feel what a thrill it is to see a horse you have bred and raised win a significant race, there would be more people in the horse business.

Just past the federal hospital on Spurr Road, watch on the left for a significant mansion beyond a significant gate. That's **Vinery Farm,** one of the old ones, where a stallion named **Red Ransom** and others stand at stud.

Bethel Presbyterian Church

You take a left on Yarnallton and then a right on Bethel Road, and come shortly to another of the area's venerable Presbyterian churches. This one was erected in 1847, but presumably took the site of an early structure, because graves there date to 1812 and 1818. It is relaxing to wander among the stones in such a churchyard and read the inscriptions, wondering about lives in long ago times.

Bethel becomes Moores Mill Road after it crosses U.S. 62 a couple of miles past the Bethel Church, and past interesting houses and beautiful country. On the right just after the road changes its name is **William R. Buster's Audubon Farm,** a thoroughbred nursery.

The Audubon residence and a nearby spring house were built about 1790. The farm once produced Aberdeen-Angus cattle from imported stock.

Equus Run Vineyards

Moore's Mill Road passes Cane Run Road a ways past Audubon Farm, and we'll eventually want to go that way. But first, there's the winery to explore around the corner and across South Elkhorn Creek.

Equus Run Vineyards is not a bad place to have a picnic, and the management encourages you to bring along a lunch. It offers sample wines in its tasting room as well as a welcome to its grounds.

The winery is open year-round, with winter hours 11 a.m. to 5 p.m. Tuesday through Saturday. In summer, the hours are the same as in winter from Tuesday through Thursday. But Friday and Saturday hours are different between March 31 and October 31, when they are 11 a.m. to 7 p.m.

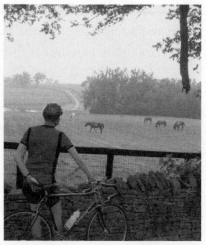

Dave McGinty, pausing to check out some horses over a stone wall on Bethel Road not far from Equus Vineyards.

Backtrack a Bit

From the winery you head back down Moores Mill Road to that intersection with Cane Run Road, turn left and ride under the interstate highway. That's **Glencrest Farm**, a full-service Thoroughbred breeding, boarding and sales operation on the right just after I-64.

Turn right on Ironworks Pike, a remnant of an old War of 1812 road that moved cannon balls and other military iron from the area around Owingsville down to the river at Frankfort, to be shipped to General Jackson down in New Orleans.

Be careful. Ironworks has become a little busy in recent years. But it's ridable in stretches, and will become somewhat less busy as soon as you re-cross U.S 62 in less than a mile.

On the way, though, notice the historic marker at the former home of **George W. Johnson**, who was the first Confederate Governor of Kentucky. He was named governor in 1861 and had to hightail it to Bowling Green because the CSA army was weak around here. He fought as a private at Shiloh the next year and was mortally wounded. He's buried near here.

On to Yarnallton

Beyond U.S. 62 you'll pass **Peninsula Farm**, which offers breeding, boarding and sales prep of Standardbred horses. Their top stallion has the un-workmanlike name of **Jenna's Beach Boy**, but he won almost $2 million when he was racing.

You come up on Yarnallton Road in a bit, and it should sound familiar. That's the way back to Spurr Road and the start. You jog around a little bit where Hamilton Lane comes in from the right about a mile after you reach Yarnallton

You'll pass **War Horse Place** along there. It's a broodmare boarding farm, for a limited number of mares, its advertising says. Breeders from other parts of the country bring mares to Kentucky to be bred to its great stallions, and then they often stay around for a while at broodmare places.

You'll cross the Interstate again and reach Spurr Road, to retrace your route back to the soccer complex.

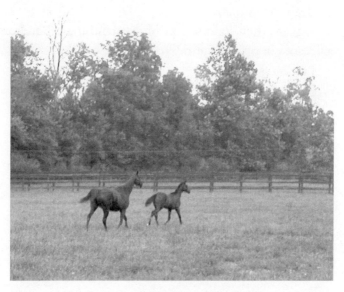

A mare and foal on a Bethel Road horse farm.

Route Sheet

0.0	Soccer complex parking lot, Masterso2n Station Park, right on the park road
0.5	Right on Shamrock Road, past stables
0.9	Bear left on Shamrock.
1.3	Left on Spurr Road
2.1	Warden's impressive house on left
3.2	Left on Yarnallton Road
3.7	Right on Bethel Road
4.8	Bethel Presbyterian Church
4.9	Left to continue on Bethel, passing Falconwood
6.0	Cross U.S. 62. Continue on Moores Mill Road.
7.5	Pass Cane Run Road on right. Stay on Moores Mill.
7.9	Winery. Turn around.
8.4	Left on Cane Run
10.0	Right on Ironworks Pike
10.9	Confederate Governor historic sign
11.8	Cross U.S. 62.
14.9	Right on Yarnallton
16.2	Jog left, then right to stay on Yarnallton as Hamilton Lane comes in on the right. Cross I-64.
17.6	Left on Spurr
19.5	Right on Shamrock
20.3	Left on park road
20.8	Back at parking lot

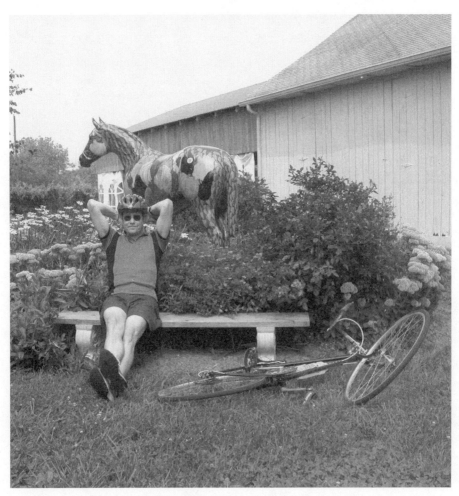

Dave McGinty stretching his legs at Equus Vineyards, on a bench near a painted horse entitled Vegetariat.

Big Sink Road Ride

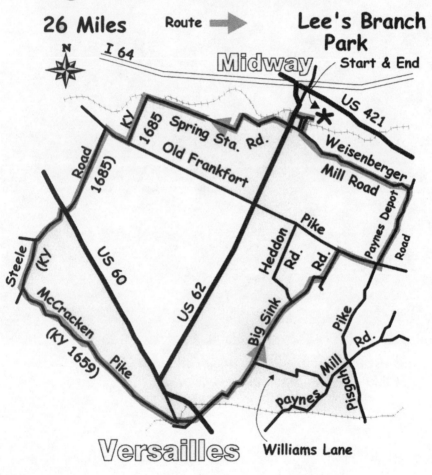

26 Miles Route ➡ **Lee's Branch Park**
Start & End

3

Big Sink Ride

Twenty-six miles. Moderate hills. Some traffic in Midway and Versailles, otherwise, little. Start at Lee's Branch Park at the end of Dudley Street in Midway, Ky. From I-64, about 10 miles west of Lexington, take exit 65. Follow U.S. 62 to Main Street, turn east, jog left on Gratz Street, and take Dudley right to the park.

This is another of my favorite "Taste of Bluegrass" rides. It just seems to have everything. It starts in **Midway,** a great little Bluegrass town, goes through Versailles, another one, and passes beautiful horse farms and historic churches and other structures all along the way. It's a reasonable length for novice riders, and can be combined with several other rides in the book for people who want a little more distance.

After I moved from Lexington to Louisville and started riding with the **Louisville Bicycle Club,** whenever friends wanted a good ride in the Bluegrass, this is the one I would take them on. One November day I took my friends **Martha Elson** and **Bill Pike** on this ride, and we were all charmed to hear the same Christmas carol on loudspeakers up and down Main Street in Midway.

Start at Midway's **Lee's Branch Memorial Park** and head up Dudley Street to jog left on Gratz Street and right on Main Street. The presence of the railroad track down the middle of Main Street gives you a hint about how Midway got started back in 1835. It was the midway point on the newly-organized Lexington and Ohio Railroad Co.'s line between Frankfort and Lexington. The railroad bought **John Francisco's** farm and laid out a town.

John Hunt Morgan

Confederate raider **John Hunt Morgan** came through here in July, 1862, and had the track torn up when he heard a union troop train from **Frankfort** was headed this way. The train went back. Then Morgan got on the telegraph and tried to coax another union train over from Lexington. But it backed off, too. So Morgan moved on to **Georgetown.**

Morgan was from Lexington. When Kentucky gave up its neutrality in the Civil War and declared itself for the union, Morgan slipped out of town at the head of a rifle company he'd organized before the war. He ultimately became a confederate brigadier general and hero, and did a lot of raiding around the state.

But he was under suspension from his command when he was killed at **Greenville, Tenn.**, on September 10, 1864. A court of inquiry into reports of robbery and looting on his last raid was pending.

Morgan's name must appear on more Kentucky historical markers than any other human being.

To the Countryside

Turn left on U.S. 62 at the head of Main Street, and pass a lot of picturesque and historic buildings. Turn right on West Stephens Street, and you'll soon find yourself out in the countryside on Spring Station Road. It winds around a bit to get out to the community of Spring Station, and then crosses the track and heads out for **Old Frankfort Pike.** There are some nice stone walls along the way.

Old Frankfort Pike runs between Lexington and Frankfort, and is one of Kentucky's best-known scenic byways. Traffic on it has become a bit heavy for cycling in recent years, but sections of it are still pretty ridable.

We won't be on it long here. But you should note that, on the left, as we travel west to a left turn on Steele Road, is a chunk of **Airdrie Stud,** the farm of former Kentucky Governor **Brereton C. Jones.** He was governor from 1991 to 1995. Some think he might be again one day.

Part of the farm is on land that once was **Woodburn Stud,** home of **Lexington,** a 19th century stallion whose years as the top Thoroughbred stud have never been surpassed, and of five 19th century Kentucky Derby Winners. It is, Jones says, "in fact the birthplace of Kentucky's Thoroughbred industry."

Sheikh Maktoum bin Rashid al Maktoum

Up Steele Road a bit we come to **Gainesborough Farm**, founded in 1984 by the above-named Sheikh, who is vice president and prime minister of the **United Arab Emirates**, and ruler of **Dubai**. The place is fantastic. It looks like a Bluegrass equivalent of something out of the Arabian Nights.

The barns are huge and beautiful. The grounds are immaculate. On the Bluegrass club's Horsey Hundred ride, I have seen riders from places like Nebraska standing astride their bicycles and just looking at Gainesborough Farm, unwilling to push on.

Sheikh Maktoum and his brother, **Sheikh Mohammed bin Rashid al Maktoum**, crown prince of Dubai and Defense Minister of the UAE, are frequent bidders of large sums at Keeneland horse sales. They arrive at Bluegrass Field across U.S. 60 from the race track in separate Boeing 747 airplanes, which sit there, huge, while they are at the sales.

Gulp

When the September 11 attacks occurred in New York, I happened to be at the Keeneland September yearling sale, filling in for **Kirsten Haukebo**, who was *The Courier-Journal's* business news horse writer. I wasn't feeling too sure of my ground anyway, and didn't need a real tough task. But Sheikh Mohammed was right there in the crowd—a very prominent Islamic leader whose views on the event would no doubt interest our readers.

He moved around the sales pavilion and viewing area openly, but he was sort of inside a group of formidable looking men. Plus, there was the fact that he was just very rich, and probably very powerful. On the plus side, he was wearing a t-shirt, jeans, and a pair of sneakers. I swallowed hard and went after him. I caught him by lurking at a narrow place where his entourage had to go single file.

He was very gracious. It wasn't an assault on America, he said, but an attack on all mankind, to be condemned by all reasonable people. Good answer.

There's More

You clear Gainesborough and cross U.S. 60 to find yourself riding through **Diamond A Farms**, with barns on both sides of the road that look every bit as glamorous as those of the Maktoums. On one stretch of road, you're in a place where you can see only plank fences, green, rolling pastures, and improbable, cupola-topped barns in every direction as far as your eye can reach.

Take a left to stay on Steele Road, and then another when you drop down along side Glenn's Creek. Notice the picturesque old **Glen's Creek Baptist Church** in the trees just beyond the intersection. But don't ask me to explain the discrepancy in the spelling.

You find yourself on McCracken Pike, headed for Versailles. On the left along there you pass a chunk of **Ashford Stud,** where Derby Winners **Fusaichi Pegasus** and **Thunder Gulch**, and a bunch of other noted stallions, stand at stud. It costs $125,000 to have your mare bred to Fusaichi, the 2000 Derby winner. Thunder Gulch, who won in 1995, can be had for $65,000.

Versailles

As you ride into Versailles you'll be on Maple Street, and if you listen closely, you might hear an old man's voice singing **"My Old Kentucky Home."** You'll be passing the home of the late A.B. "Happy" Chandler, who was twice Kentucky governor, and who also served in the U.S. Senate. He also was the national commissioner of baseball who presided over **Jackie Robinson's** move into the major leagues in 1947.

Happy was an old populist, and he used to sing the state song in public whenever anybody would let him.

When you cross U.S. 60 in Versailles, McCracken Pike becomes Broadway. There are a number of places to grab a sandwich or a cold drink in Versailles, and one of them, **Huff's Grocery and Deli,** is right on your way, on the left just after you turn left on Douglas Avenue.

Huff's is famous for its Mom's Meatloaf sandwich, which cost $2.99 when I was there in 2003. It's open from 8 a.m. to 4 p.m. every day. It has a public rest room.

Big Sink Road

Continue on Douglas across U.S. 60 again and some railroad tracks, and you'll find yourself on the Big Sink Road. I've always loved that name. I love the road, too. It used to be toward the end of my ride when I'd pedal from Louisville down to Georgetown for the Horsey Hundred in years gone by. I always felt great when I got to Big Sink Road.

As Big Sink approaches Old Frankfort Pike, you'll pass the van entrance to Three Chimneys Farm, where **Seattle Slew** used to stand. He was the only undefeated Triple Crown winner. He died in 2002. **Silver Charm,** another Derby winner and the third leading money winner in racing history, as this book was being written, was still at stud there. He sold for $16,500 as a yearling, and won $6,941,369 before retiring to stud.

The Old Mill

You go right on Old Frankfort Pike, and ride about a mile down to Paynes Depot Road. That takes you a couple of miles on down to Weisenberger Mill Road, where you will turn left. But first, you might detour about a tenth of a mile to the right to **Weisenberger Mill**, where you can stand on a bridge and watch **South Elkhorn Creek** flow past the mill.

There's no water wheel, because the creek turns a couple of turbines to grind grain, as it has since the early 1800s. "It's more efficient," Phil Weisenberger told me, though he conceded that turbines are less picturesque than water wheels. Phil is the fifth generation of the family that has operated the mill since 1865.

He said the existing building was built in 1913. His son, Mack, runs the mill now, with help from his own son, Philip, who was in his late 20s as this was written. You can buy an assortment of milled grains at the mill, including such specialty items as spoon bread and hush puppy mix, but there are no tours anymore.

"We haven't had tours since OSHA came into being," Phil Weisenberger said. "Our lawyers don't want us to take the risk."

Midway College

Retracing your steps on Weisenberger Mill Road past Paynes Depot Road takes you another three miles or so into Midway, passing Midway

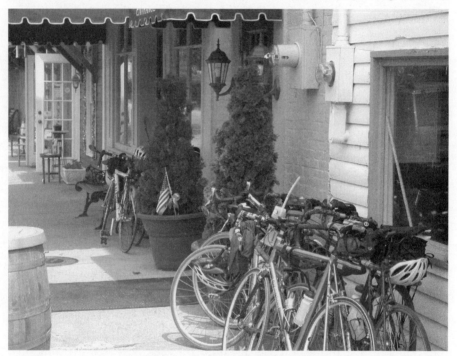

Bikes stack up outside a Midway eatery during the Horsey Hundred

College just before you get into town. Midway is a liberal arts school that bills itself as Kentucky's only college for women. It was founded in 1847 to prepare financially disadvantaged young women as teachers, and it was originally called the **Kentucky Female Orphan School.**

It now trains women for careers in nursing, as paralegals, and in equine management. Early in its history, the Horsey Hundred bicycle ride used Midway College as a place to put riders overnight, and I have fond memories of the grounds there. The ride soon got too big for Midway College though, and now uses nearby Georgetown College.

Turn right on South Brand Street, and then take another right on Dudley, back into the park.

Route Sheet

0.0	Leave Lee's Branch Memorial Park on Dudley Street.
0.3	Left on Gratz, then right on E. Main
0.4	Left on U.S. 62
1.5	Right on W. Stephens Street (becomes Spring Station Road)
4.3	Left on KY 1685
5.3	Right on Old Frankfort Pike
5.9	Left on Steele Road (KY 1685)
7.9	Cross U.S. 60.
8.9	Follow Steele Road left.
10.0	Left on McCracken Pike (KY 1659)
14.6	Cross U.S. 60 onto Broadway.
14.9	Left on Douglas Street
15.0	Cross U.S. 60. Douglas becomes Big Sink Road.
16.8	Pass Williams Lane on right.
20.0	Right on Old Frankfort Pike
20.9	Left on Paynes Depot Road
22.7	Left on Weisenberger Mill Road
25.6	Right on S. Brand Street
25.8	Right on Dudley Street into park

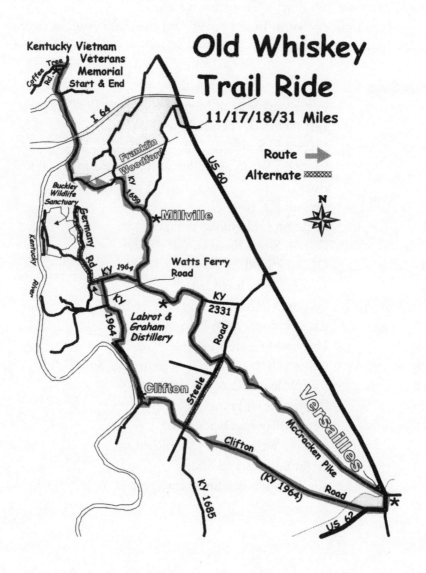

4

Old Whiskey Trail Ride

> *Rides varying in length from 11 to 31 miles. Some hills, depending on route choice. Moderate traffic. Start at Kentucky Vietnam Veterans Memorial in Frankfort. From I-64 east of Frankfort, take Exit 58, U.S. 60 west. Go 1.2 miles toward town and on 60, then turn left on KY 676 and follow it to Coffee Tree Road. Look for Memorial signs.*

This ride starts in **Frankfort** and follows a winding path past a couple of old distilleries that were very significant in the development of bourbon whiskey, which—with fast horses and beautiful women—is at the top of the list of things that make Kentucky famous. It passes a working craft distillery, where a premium bourbon is painstakingly produced, and where a rider can pause to learn a good deal about the history and lore of the amber elixir.

It passes through some very nice countryside to the pleasant Bourbon County seat of Versailles, and winds its way back. A couple of shorter rides are pointed out, for riders who are just getting their cranking legs, or have time only for a short jaunt. One of those actually starts in Versailles and comes back toward Frankfort, before looping around to finish back in Versailles.

Engineering Marvel

The longer, main, ride starts on a bit of a somber note at the **Kentucky Vietnam Veterans Memorial**, which sits high on a hill overlooking the **Kentucky Capitol** in Frankfort. In a very unique way, it honors about 1,100 Kentucky soldiers who died in the Vietnam War.

Their names are all carved into granite blocks arrayed on a plaza that makes up a huge sundial. The blocks and the gnomon, or pointer, are arranged in such a way that the shadow of the gnomon touches the name of each soldier on the anniversary of his death in the war.

The effect, as **Charles K. Aked** of the **British Sundial Society** has noted, is that the whole million-plus-dollar memorial stands for the memory of a single person at a particular moment. It's a great idea that was more easily voiced than realized.

Computer Aided Design

The monument was the brain child of **Helm Roberts**, a Lexington architect and planner who knew about naval charts that would tell where the sun is at any given time of day. He figured that meant you also could tell where its shadow would be.

He worked on the idea for a history-oriented sundial in Lexington in 1974, but that project never got off the ground. He dusted the theory off and presented it to the competition committee for the veterans memorial when it asked for ideas in 1987. The committee loved it, and chose it unanimously, but expressed worry that it might not work.

Actually, Roberts told me, "it turned out to be more difficult than I thought it would be." But he found a computer aided design program to do some of the hard work, and eventually it all worked out just as he'd thought it would.

Tons of Granite

And an amazing thing it is. The plaza floor is made of dozens of slabs of granite, 10 feet by three feet and 1,500 pounds on average, 215 tons in all. They sit on 800 concrete piers. A temporary gnomon was set up while the design was still underway to make sure the computer knew what it was talking about. But ultimately the stones were all cut and the names carved at a different location, then brought to the site, where they fit perfectly. And worked.

As is the case with the **Vietnam Memorial** in Washington, people come to the Frankfort site and leave poems, flowers, beer cans, boots, all sorts of tribute to those who sacrificed. The items are gathered up and stored in a history museum.

Roberts likes to take children to the site to talk to them about history and war, and about careful measurement and construction. One thing they learn there, he said, is what a cubit is. The gnomon, a 3/16-inch stainless steel plate, is 10 cubits high. A cubit is 18 inches, so that's 15 feet to you and me.

The Main Ride

The roads on this ride offer a number of possibilities, and I'll discuss some of them in a moment. But first, this is how I first envisioned the ride —as a nice, medium-length ride that combines whiskey lore with horse farms, a couple of quaint villages, a nice little country town, and a lot of good, rich Kentucky countryside.

Start by heading down Coffee Tree Road to KY 1659, and duck down along the **Kentucky River.** Before long, you'll come to a couple of old distillery properties—**Old Crow** and **Old Taylor.** They don't distill whiskey there anymore, but they store some.

The Old Crow brand was named for **James Christopher Crow**, who worked at the **Elijah Pepper** distillery, which is still in operation as **LeBrot & Graham Distillery** up the road a bit. Crow introduced scientific principles and instruments to the creation of bourbon, making it the smooth and uniform product we know today.

The **Old Taylor** brand was named for **Col. Edmund Taylor**, who owned the Pepper distillery for a while, too. So a stop at Lebrot and Graham will put you in touch with the foundations of bourbon.

First, There's Millville

Once you pass the old distilleries, you start encountering the strung-out village of **Millville.** They pitch a lot of horseshoes here. You can get a cold drink or a sandwich—or a hot meal—at the **Old Millville Store and**

Grill, which operates on a split shift. It's open from 7 a.m. to 2 p.m. and from 5 p.m. to midnight Monday through Friday. Hours on Saturday are 2 p.m. to midnight, and the store is closed on Sunday.

Pedal on past the store and past KY 1964, which comes in on the right, and you'll soon find yourself at the previously-mentioned LeBrot & Graham distillery. It's a good place to grab a sandwich as well as to learn about bourbon.

You can wander around in the distillery's visitor center, reading about whiskey history, and there's a free hour-and-a-quarter tour led by engaging and knowledgeable tour guides.

Whiskey People

Lebrot & Graham is owned by Louisville-based **Brown-Forman Corporation**, maker and marketer of such whiskeys as **Jack Daniels** and **Old Forester**. It could be argued that Lebrot & Graham is that huge company's answer to the success of **Maker's Mark,** which has a similarly small and historic distillery making premium bourbon down near **Loretto**, Ky. Each claims to be the smallest and oldest.

But it is a historic place. Elijah Pepper started making whiskey in Versailles in 1797, and moved out here on Glenn's Creek in 1812. His house, a log cabin, is still here. Lebrot & Graham bought the place in 1878, and owned it into the 1940s. Their tenure was interrupted by prohibition, though, and when Brown-Forman bought out the Lebrots, it was largely to get the 30,000 barrels of whiskey that had been stored here through that trying period for distillers.

Brown-Forman moth-balled the place in 1972, and revived it in 1994 for the purpose of "hand-crafting" its Woodford Reserve brand. Which, I have to say, is very good whiskey.

The distillery is open from 9 a.m. to 5 p.m. Tuesday through Saturday, and 12:30 to 4:30 on Sunday. Tour times weekdays are at 10 and 11 a.m., and 1, 2, and 3 p.m. On Sundays, only the three afternoon tours are offered. Visitors must be of drinking age to enter the distillery.

Scenic McCracken Pike

Beyond the distillery, you stay on KY 1659 past Steele Road, onto McCracken Pike, which takes you into Versailles. It's a very nice ride.

Versailles is perhaps best known as the home of A.B. "Happy" Chandler, a colorful Kentucky politician, who was governor twice and U.S. Senator once. He's buried over by the Pisgah Presbyterian Church. McCracken Pike becomes Maple Street as it enters Versailles, and if you watch on the left as you pedal into town, you'll see Happy's mail box.

Turn right at Main Street, which is also U.S. 60. Be careful. There will be some traffic.

If it happens to be lunch time, or if you happen to be hungry even if it's not, you should be aware that right there on Main Street, across from the Court House, is **Debbie's Café**, owned by **Debbie Durrum** and her mother, **Barbara Durrum**.

It's a breakfast and lunch operation, open from 6 a.m. to 2 p.m. every day except Sunday, when it's closed. It offers home cooking, a full menu with vegetables of several kinds and three or four meats. There also are the usual hamburgers, cheeseburgers and such. And interesting people eat there.

Turn right again at Morgan Street, which is also U.S. 62, and will shortly become Clifton Road. You can get soft drinks or snacks at the Neighborhood Grocery on Clifton just after U.S. 62 goes off to the left. But the store does not offer sandwiches, and it has no public rest room.

Down, Down, Down to Clifton

You ride out Clifton Road past a right turn at Steele Road, and after a bit find yourself in a pretty steep, twisty downhill, as the road descends into the river bottom. For the moment, don't even think about the possibility that if the road goes down there, somewhere it has to come up. Be careful.

On your left once you arrive at the bottom is **Clifton**, which once was a weekend and holiday community. With the improvement of roads, though, people moved down there permanently, and now most are full-time residents.

There's an intriguing stone smoke stack on the river bank about half way through the town, visible from Old Clifton Road, if you want to take a slight detour. It stands there alone, the attached buildings having long since burned away from it. **Lorraine Brandenburg**, at the **Woodford County Historical Society**, told me it was a distillery called the **J.H. Frazier Co.** in 1905.

Gary Jones at the Woodford County Chamber of Commerce said it later functioned as a mill, and still later as a residence.

About That Climb

Now you can start thinking about the likelihood that having enjoyed a long downhill into the river valley, you might expect to climb a bit to get out. In truth, the hill you'll soon come to is about a mile long, and not as steep as some I've seen. The thing to do is put the old derailleur in stump puller gear, and grind away. You'll be up before you know it, and in a position to tell your friends that you took the scenic route down to the river, and back up.

A ways after you clear the top of the hill, you hang a right where Watts Ferry Road comes in, and a left back on Kentucky 1659. Then just retrace your trail back to the memorial, with a possible stop at the Millville store for a cold Ale-8-One.

A Tale of Many Rides

While I was going over the map for this ride, ever mindful that I needed short rides for beginners, it occurred to me that there are a number of possibilities here. First I thought I should offer an alternative to the main route for people who don't necessarily want an invigorating climb out of the Kentucky River Valley north of Clifton. So I threw in a shortcut across Steele Road on the way back.

Then I started slicing and dicing until my wife **Suzanne's** eyes glazed over as I described the possibilities. Suffice it to say there are several possible rides here, and here are a couple more of them:

Birds and Wildflowers

One good possibility is a ride just down to the **Buckley Wildlife Sanctuary** and back, taking in the charm of the woodsy area along the river bank and through scenic Millville. If you do that ride, which is about 17.6 miles round trip, you might consider using a set of panniers, with a pair of hiking shoes in one and a picnic lunch in the other.

Just take Coffee Tree Road out of the memorial, take a right on KY 1659, and follow it along the river and past the old distilleries and turn right again on KY 1964. You'll pick up the Buckley Sanctuary signs.

Buckley is a natural wonder, with birds, mammals and wildflowers in abundance, a nice place to sit in the bird blind for a while, or to take a short hike. There also are good places to picnic. The sanctuary is open Wednesday through Friday from 9 a.m. to 5 p.m., and from 9 to 6 on Saturday and Sunday.

It's closed Mondays, Tuesdays and holidays, and for the entire months of January and February. Regular admission is $3 if you're over 16 and $2 if you're under. It can be more for special events.

A Short Sashay into the Bluegrass

Or, for a shorter trip with perhaps fewer hills, one could just do the Versailles to Steele Road portion of the main ride. That would be 11.2 miles. Throw in a trip to Lebrot & Graham Distillery, and it grows to almost 17.

To do that ride, you'd want to start at the **Versailles Presbyterian Church**, at 130 N. Main St. in Versailles, which is on U.S. 60 12 miles east of Frankfort. Just follow U.S. 60 into town, rather than taking the bypass, and you'll be on Main Street. Versailles Presbyterian is right across the street from the **Woodford County Chamber of Commerce**, where people would be glad to tell you about Woodford County's other offerings.

You take a right out of the church parking lot and go a couple of tenths of a mile up to a left turn on Maple Street. That becomes McCracken Pike, or KY 1659. Take that out to Steele Road, take a left and ride across to Clifton Road, and pedal back into Versailles and the church.

Or, vice versa. There are a lot of good Kentucky farms of all types to see along the way. To add the distillery, don't take the left on Steele Road. Just stay on KY 1659 until you get to it. It's almost three miles. Then turn around, take a right on Steele and follow the ride sheet.

Route Sheet

0.0	Vietnam Veterans Memorial, left on Coffee Tree Road
0.3	Right on Glenn's Creek Road, KY 1659
3.7	Old Crow warehouses
4.3	Old Taylor properties
5.7	Old Millville Store & Grill
6.7	Pass KY 1964.
7.5	Lebrot & Graham Distillery
10.2	Cross Steele Road.
14.8	Right on Main Street, in Versailles
15.1	Left on Morgan Street, U.S. 62
15.5	Straight on Clifton Pike (KY 1964) Neighborhood Grocery on the left.
19.7	Pass Steele Road. (Note: this is where you turn right if you want to avoid the ride down to — and climb out of — the river. It's 1.6 miles back to KY 1659, where you'll go left just past the old church, to retrace the route back to Frankfort. The whole trip is 30.4 miles if you take that route.)
20.1	Start down a long, twisty hill to the river. Be careful. There are some sharp turns.
21.1	Bear right on KY 1964. Pass the little community of Clifton, and start climbing.
24.1	Right to stay on 1964. (Left is Watts Ferry Road, which goes to Buckley Sanctuary.)
24.9	Left on KY 1659
25.9	Old Millville Store
30.6	Left onto Coffeetree Road
30.9	Back at Parking Lot

Buckley Sanctuary Short Route

0.0	Vietnam Veterans Memorial, left on Coffee Tree Road
0.3	Right on Glenn's Creek Road, KY 1659
3.7	Old Crow warehouses
4.3	Old Taylor properties
5.7	Old Millville Store & Grill
6.7	Right on KY 1964
7.6	Stay straight on Watts Ferry Road.
7.8	Right on Germany Road
8.8	Sanctuary entrance. Turn around.
9.8	Left on Watts Ferry.
10.0	Straight on KY 1964
10.9	Left on KY 1694
11.9	Old Millville Store
17.3	Left on Coffee Tree
17.6	Back at memorial

Versailles Short Ride

0.0	Versailles Presbyterian Church Parking Lot. Right on Main Street
0.2	Left on Elm Street (McCracken Pike, KY 1659)
4.8	Pass Steele Road (or turn left if you want to bypass the distillery. This short ride is 11.2 miles if you do that.)
7.6	Lebrot and Graham. Turn around
10.5	Right on Steele Road
12.2	Left on Clifton Pike (KY 1964)
16.3	Neighborhood Grocery on right
16.7	Left on Main Street
16.9	Back at church

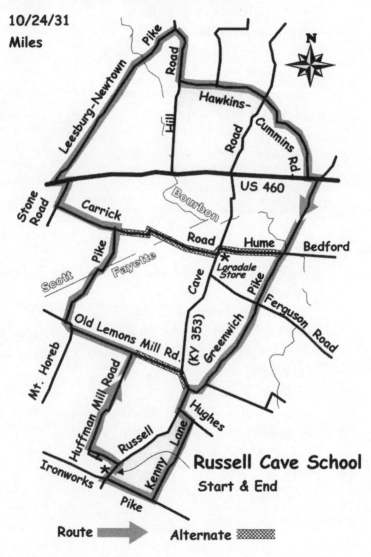

Jot 'Em Down Ride

10/24/31
Miles

Russell Cave School
Start & End

Route ➡️   Alternate ▨

5

Jot 'Em Down Ride

Three routes, of 10, 23 and 31 miles. Moderate hills.
Some traffic on Ironworks Pike. Start at Russell Cave Elementary
school, a tenth of a mile north of Ironworks Pike at Russell
Cave Road. Take Exit 120 from I-75 just north of Lexington and go
southwest on Ironworks Pike for five miles.

This ride is like the Keeneland ride in that it skirts some of the most famous horse farms in the Bluegrass, and wanders along some of the most beautiful agricultural land in the country.

In my continuing effort to be all things to all people, I offer you here three options to fit your cycling needs. If you are new to riding or don't have much time, you might consider option A, which is about 10 miles long. Option B, which I'll call medium, is about 23 miles long.

And option C, which I'll call the main ride, is slightly more medium, at about 31 miles. And for those of you to whom a 30-mile ride is hardly worth getting out of the house for, I invite you to combine this with another ride, say Paris-Beth-Paris, or Tour de France. Or hey, both.

A School Start

I call all three the Jot 'Em Down Ride because they start near a famous old Bluegrass country store, about which I'll have more to say later. There's not much parking at Jot 'Em Down, though, and there's plenty at Russell Cave Elementary School, which is about a tenth of a mile north on Russell Cave Road. So the Bluegrass club starts a lot of rides there.

59

Actually, it's sort of an interesting school. It's actually called **Russell Cave Model Magnet Elementary School**, and it's a partnership between **Fayette County Public Schools** and **Transylvania University** in Lexington.

It started as a one-room country school sometime before 1900 on the nearby **Mt. Brilliant Farm**. In its present configuration, it offers the usual reading, writing and arithmetic, and it has special programs for learning disorders, special education, gifted education, and band and orchestra.

Report of a Pistol, Flash of a Knife

You ride a short distance up Russell Cave Road from the school, and turn right on Huffman Mill Pike. On your right at that point is a corner of Mt. Brilliant Farm, which dates from 1774 and once was owned by **James Ben Ali Haggin**, a storied rich person.

The farm is the site of **Russell Cave**, a cavern near which there was many a political gathering during the 19th century. It was the site of emancipationist **Cassius M. Clay**'s famous 1843 gun and knife fight with **Samuel M. Brown**.

Clay was a Kentucky native from down by **Richmond**, who went off to Yale College and came back with funny ideas against slavery. He was outspoken, and widely hated in slave-holding Kentucky. Brown attacked him with a pistol during a debate at the cave, aiming at his heart at close range. The shot didn't slow the obstreperous Clay down much, though, and he carved Brown up pretty well with his Bowie knife.

It turned out the bullet had been deflected by the silver lining of the knife's sheath, which Clay kept strapped across his chest. Clay was charged with mayhem, but he got off on self defense. He had a good lawyer: his cousin, **Henry Clay.**

Cassius Clay went on to play an important part in **Abraham Lincoln**'s administration. There's more about him on the White Hall Ride.

Tumbling Mansions

The previously mentioned Haggin, whose forebears included a central Kentucky pioneer and an expatriated Turk, bought Mt. Brilliant along with a bunch of other farms around here in the late 1800s and early 1900s. He had gone out to the gold fields of California and made a lot of money as a lawyer, and then in mining. Later he hooked up with such people as **Marcus Daly** and **Sen. George Hearst,** father of **William Randolph,** in copper mines in **Montana** and **Peru.**

He got very rich, and he built a huge mansion, said to rival the **Biltmore Hotel** in New York, on the old **Elmendorf Farm** a ways down Ironworks Pike. It was all columns and marble, and Haggin even had a rail spur run to it, to bring in fancy guests. But the mansion is probably most famous for lasting only from 1902 to 1929. Haggin died, and a new, also rich, owner, **Joseph Widener,** thought the place was too expensive to keep up.

Stay with me here. This is all going somewhere. The Russell family, for whom the cave, the road and the school are named, sold Mt. Brilliant in 1832, and it passed through various hands, including Haggin's, until it ended up with the current owner, **Greg Goodman,** a rich person from Houston.

Goodman caused a flap a couple of years ago in preservation-minded Fayette County by proposing to tear down another mansion on the farm, one that still had some parts of an old 1792 Russell house inside it somewhere. He listened to the hue and cry, but insisted that restoration would be too expensive and impractical. And he tore it down, in late 2002.

But All is Not Lost

All that said, you should know that the cave and the site of the torn down Russell mansion all are on a part of Mt. Brilliant that you won't pass too closely, because they're on the Russell Cave Road side, where the traffic often is heavy. I tell you about them because you at least skirt the farm.

But, right on Huffman Mill Pike, just after the chunk of Mt. Brilliant, is what used to be **Man O' War Farm,** where the great Thoroughbred once lived. Goodman also bought that farm, right after he tore down the mansion. But he's not messing with anything really sacred.

He noted that the barn and breeding shed used by Man O' War were in bad shape, but said he'd rebuild them. He said he would restore the barn to the way it was when the horse of the century, last century, used it.

And Man O' War's stall, with its original door, will be left empty, Goodman said.

Also, he plans to restore the garden over at Mt. Brilliant. Mt. Brilliant, incidentally was named for the Virginia estate of **Patrick Henry**, because the first Russell was Henry's brother-in-law. Besides the unlucky mansion, the farm had beautiful gardens, and Goodman said he'd restore them - to include a vineyard, a kitchen garden full of berries, herbs and vegetables, and a formal English flower garden.

His Excellency

If you're doing the short ride, turn right at Old Lemons Mill Road, and follow the route sheet back to the school. Otherwise, turn left at Old Lemons, and head up Mt. Horeb Road, across Carrick Road, and up Stone Road to Newtown.

As you go up Mt. Horeb, you will pass the Oak Tree Division of **Lane's End Farm**, on your left. Lane's End, the main part of which is along the unfortunately busy U.S. 62 between Versailles and Old Frankfort Pike, belongs to **Will S. Farish**, who is U.S. Ambassador to Great Britain as this book is written.

He boards some horses that belong to Queen Elizabeth II of England, and one of his good friends is **U.S. President George W. Bush**. Both the queen and the president have been guests at the farm. Maybe even this part.

Downtown Newtown

One of the several pikes that radiate out of Lexington—the one, in fact, that motorists traveling from the west take into town from I-64, is called Newtown Pike. It's a very familiar road around here. From Old Lemons Mill Road we reach a chunk of Mt. Horeb Pike and Carrick and Stone roads, and we arrive at Newtown, that road's destination.

Turns out, there's not much there. If you are taking the 23-mile route, incidentally, you already will have turned right at Carrick (instead of left) and will be following that route sheet back.

You main route riders take a short chunk of U.S. 460 out of

Newtown, to Leesburg-Newtown Pike, and on up to Hill Road. It's all great riding. Hawkins-Cummins Road takes us back to another short run on U.S. 460, and then down the beautiful Greenwich Pike.

Get into the Horse Business

As I was writing this, there was a farm for sale on Greenwich, about half way down. **David and Ginger Mullins,** were selling the 113-acre **Doninga Farm**, which selling agent **Bill Justice** said is an "exceptional parcel of land."

There, in 2001, the Mullinses bred the Storm Cat filly **Platinum Heights**, which they sold at the Keeneland July Sale in 2002 for $2.8 million. She was the top-priced yearling filly of that year. I didn't ask what it would take to buy the place.

At the end of Greenwich you take a short chunk of Russell Cave Road and Hughes Lane, to Kenny Lane and back to Ironworks Pike

Unforgettable Leslie Combs II

Be careful. Ironworks Pike has become a little busy in recent years, but it's ridable for short stretches. And this is a stretch you gotta do. On your left is **Spendthrift Farm**, one of the region's most famous, former home of the great stud **Nashua**—first Thoroughbred to sell for $1 million—and of eight Derby winners during their breeding years. Spendthrift was built and operated by **Leslie Combs II**, a noted character as well as a fabled horseman.

I got to interview Combs one year leading up to Derby. I enjoyed it a lot. He put me in his car, which had a button he could push that produced the call to the post when he saw anybody he felt like tooting at. He drove me all around his farm.

He took me back to the house for lunch. We had chicken wings and consommé. There were a couple of cruets of sherry on the table, and he added some of that to his consommé. So I did, too. It was delicious.

We ate in a sort of a sunroom, with a couple of walls full of windows, and green, rolling pasture just outside. He said he served his Derby guests breakfast there. The night before, he'd have somebody dump some oats in the grass a short distance out, so that foals would be sure to cavort there in the morning sunlight.

Entertaining Royalty

Combs showed me the room where he'd entertained **Princess Margaret** of England a few years earlier. He told her he was going to make her a mint julep, he said. But he just took a silver julep cup and put a little crushed ice in it, and a sprig of mint, and filled it up with bourbon.

He watched her as she drank it. She didn't bat an eye, he said. Before long it was gone, and she handed him the cup and said, "May I have anothuh?"

Combs drove me over to a chunk he then owned of the old Elmendorf Farm, which his great-grandfather, **Daniel Swigert**, had once owned. Swigert was a well-known horseman in the late 1800s, who sold a few very good horses, and eventually his whole farm, to James B.A. Haggin.

Combs started building his own farm, Spendthrift, in 1937 with his inheritance from his grandmother, Swigert's daughter. He told me he consulted geological charts to get only land that was underlain by the right kind of limestone. He bought a chunk of old Elmendorf with other land in the area.

A Hint of Scorn

Combs also drove me past the site of Haggin's mansion, where only some columns and stone lions remain. Sometimes area horsewomen used to put up a big tent there and throw a ball after the **Bluegrass Stakes** at Keeneland. Combs told me about the marble floors and the railroad spur, and noted that it was all gone. "Nobody wanted it," he said. Haggin amassed something like 10,000 acres in the area—a feat which nobody else apparently has matched—but he still lived mostly elsewhere.

Jot 'Em Down

A short distance past Spendthrift on Ironworks Pike is Russell Cave Road, and a right turn that will take you back to Russell Cave school. But first, stop at the intersection and go into the **Jot 'Em Down Store**. It was named for a fictional store in the **Lum and Abner radio show** of the 1930s through 1950s. But this Jot 'Em Down Store's claim to fame is that it got the name from Lum and Abner themselves.

The show was about a country grocery, in fictional **Pine Ridge, Ark.**, where Lum and Abner were proprietors, and it featured their interaction with an assortment of small-town characters. The whole country listened to it.

Robie Terrell, the current owner of the store on Russell Cave, said his grandfather, Lucien Terrell, used to play checkers in his store with his brother, just as Lum and Abner did in their fictional store. The Terrells got to acting like Lum and Abner, and people started calling them that, and acting like other characters in the radio skits.

Sign Provided

The story is that **Chester "Chet" Lauck** and **Norris "Tuffy" Goff**, who played Lum and Abner, were visiting the area to look at horses in a year

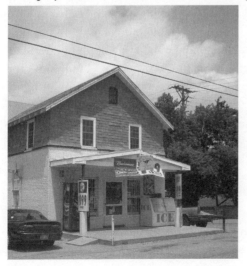

Robie Terrell seems fairly vague about. They heard about this store that was supposed to be just like the one in the radio show. So they stopped in to see for themselves, and declared it to be true. They even went to town and had a sign painted, so Terrell's Grocery could formally become the Jot 'Em Down Store.

The Jot 'Em Down Store at Ironworks and Russell Cave Pikes north of Lexington.

They make a great country ham sandwich, and have the usual snacks and soft drinks. The store's open from 9:30 a.m. to 8 p.m. every day except Sunday, when it's closed. It has public rest rooms.

Route Sheet

0.0	Leave Russell Cave School, north on Russell Cave Pike.
0.4	Left on Huffman Mill Road. Follow it around to the right.
3.6	Left on Old Lemons Mill Road
5.2	Right on Mt. Horeb Road
5.4	Right on Mt. Horeb Road
8.2	Left on Carrick Road
9.6	Right on Stone Road
10.3	Left on U.S. 460
10.6	Right on Leesburg-Newtown Pike
15.3	Right on Hill Road
16.7	Left on Hawkins-Cummins Road
18.7	Cross Russell Cave Road.
20.1	Left on U.S. 460
20.3	Right on Greenwich Pike
26.4	Left on Russell Cave
27.0	Left on Hughes Lane
27.4	Right on Kenny Lane
29.4	Right on Ironworks Pike
30.6	Jot 'em Down Store. Right on Russell Cave
30.7	Back at school

Alternate

0.0	Leave Russell Cave School, north of Russell Cave Pike.
0.4	Left on Huffman Mill Road. Follow it around to the right.
3.6	Left on Old Lemons Mill Road

5.2	Right on Mt. Horeb Road
5.4	Right on Mt. Horeb Road
8.2	Right on Carrick Road
11.0	Left on Russell Cave Road
11.2	Right on Hume Bedford Road
12.7	Right on Greenwich Pike
18.9	Left on Russell Cave
19.5	Left on Hughes Lane
19.9	Right on Kenny Lane
21.9	Right on Ironworks Pike
23.1	Jot 'em Down Store. Right on Russell Cave
23.2	Back at school

Short Jot 'Em Down Ride

0.0	Leave Russell Cave School, north of Russell Cave Pike.
0.4	Left on Huffman Mill Road. Follow it around to the right.
3.6	Right on Old Lemons Mill Road
5.0	Right on Russell Cave Road
5.4	Bear right to stay on Russell Cave.
5.9	Left on Hughes Lane
6.4	Right on Kenny Lane
8.5	Right on Ironworks Pike
9.7	Jot 'Em Down Store. Right on Russell Cave
9.8	Back at school

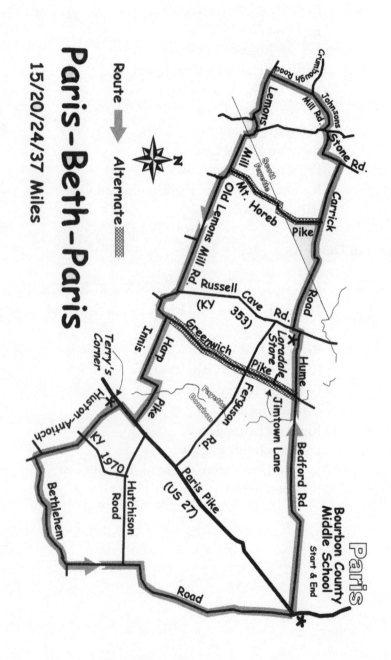

6

Paris-Beth-Paris Ride

> *Thirty-seven miles, with two alternates of 24 and 15 miles.*
> *Moderate hills and little traffic, except for a short stretch of Paris*
> *Pike. Start at Bourbon County Middle School, which is on the*
> *Paris Pike (U.S. 27) on the southwest edge of Paris, 14 miles*
> *northeast of Lexington.*

The name of this ride, like that of the Tour de France later in the book, is a sort of cyclist's joke. There's a very traditional, venerable and well-respected ride in France called **Paris-Brest-Paris**, that people have been riding since 1891. It's 750 miles long, and, while it's not a race, it is timed, and people pay close attention to how long it takes them to complete it.

In 1891, the first guy back was Charles Terront, who made it in 71 hours and 35 minutes. Now people are doing it in about 43 hours. There are elaborate rules with checkpoints and such, and you have to finish within 90 hours or they make you stop. In fact, you have to do four fairly grueling, timed rides—called brevets—before they'll even let you ride PBP.

People head out from Paris and ride as long as they can, then grab an hour or two of shuteye in a haystack somewhere, or in a van if they've thought to have somebody bring one out, and get up and ride on. Interestingly, many stop for long lunches—such as two and a half hours—because that's the way it is in France. That annoys some Americans, though **Johnny Bertrand**, of the Bluegrass Cycling Club, considers that part of the fun.

All in all, PBP, which is staged every four years, the latest in 2003, is a very big deal. It is given credit as the inspiration both for the modern Olympics and for the Tour de France. People who do PBP are looked on with awe. I read an account by an American woman who said a French bike shop did free repairs on her bike when they heard she was headed for Paris-Brest-Paris.

Pale Imitation

Like Paris-Brest-Paris, Paris-Beth-Paris—the ride you are about to embark upon here—starts and ends in Paris. From there, the similarities diverge quite a bit. For one thing, it's a whole different Paris. For another, you can probably do at least the short version of this ride in the time it takes some of those Paris-Brest-Paris people to do lunch.

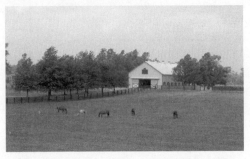

A horse pasture on Home Bedford Road, west of Paris

I've ridden across Iowa a couple of times as part of the big rolling party called RAGBRAI —the Register's Great Bicycle Ride Across Iowa—but I've never attempted even one of the brevets for PBP. Or aspired to. But I do admire people who do.

For that reason, and because this ride leaves Paris and eventually uses a stretch of Bethlehem Road before it gets back to Paris, I call this ride what I do. Plus—and this is a special bonus—it goes by the home of Johnny Bertrand, a legend in his own time who sets up the brevets for riders in Kentucky and nearby states.

Go Johnny Go

Johnny has traveled far and seen much on his bicycle, and he is revered, and deferred to, by bushwhackers and long-riders in both the Bluegrass and Louisville clubs, and no doubt others as well. He is the man who knows the roads, and he isn't reluctant to get out and ride long distances on them.

He has been organizing the PBP brevets for Kentucky since 1987. He also has mapped out several routes across Kentucky, long-ways and short-ways. And he has participated in every PBP since 1983, when he finished in

83 hours. As this was being written, he was in France riding his sixth PBP.

People who ride Paris-Brest-Paris are called "randonneurs," to distinguish them from racers like Lance Armstrong. They are people who ride hard, for long distances, for fun, though with serious enough intent to be timed. Johnny is a randonneur par excellence. You'll pass his place on Carrick Road a bit east of its intersection with Mt. Horeb Pike, on the north side.

The Alternatives

The main version of this ride is about 37 miles, going out from the **Bourbon Middle School** on Paris Pike in Paris, heading out Hume Bedford and Carrick roads, and turning south on Stone, Johnsons Mill and Crumbaugh roads. Then it follows Lemons Mill and Old Lemons Mill back to Harp Innis Pike and Paris Pike.

Paris Pike is U.S. 27, a beautiful road that goes from Lexington to Paris, which as this is written, is getting an extensive renovation intended to widen it to four lanes without ruining the beauty of the trees, stone walls and venerable mansions that have made it famous.

It's not much fun to ride on Paris Pike, because of the traffic. But short stretches are manageable, especially in those areas where the new lanes are in place. So you ride a short distance toward Lexington on Paris Pike. Be careful. Then cut left onto Huston-Antioch Road and take it down to Bethlehem road, which takes you back to Paris, in addition to giving this ride its inside humor name.

Shorter, But Just as Sweet

If you don't want even to pretend that you're training for PBP, you can take a 24-mile option by turning south when you get to Greenwich Pike, and taking Harp Innis Pike from there. Or, you can do just 15 miles by starting at the **Jimtown First Baptist Church**, just off Greenwich Pike on Jimtown Lane, and looping around Greenwich, Old Lemon's Mill, Mt. Horeb, and Carrick.

There's even a 20-mile option if you start at Jimtown, down Greenwich and all the way to Crumbaugh on Old Lemons Mill and Lemons

Mill, then follow the route back to Jimtown.

The Food

There is a store on this route, and a restaurant. **The Loradale Grocery** is on the short chunk of Russell Cave Pike that you take between Hume Bedford and Carrick roads. **Terry's Corner** restaurant is at the end of

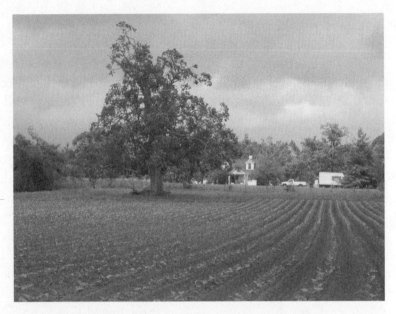

Burley tobacco plants getting started on Carrick Road, north of Lexington.

the short chunk of Paris Pike, right where you turn onto Huston-Antioch.

The Loradale store has the usual snacks and soft drinks, and they make sandwiches there. Plus, there's a pool hall. Ride up on your Litespeed with a pool cue in a leather satchel and I guarantee they'll be impressed. There is a public rest room, in the pool hall.

Terry's Corner sounds kind of fancy. It was closed when I passed through there, but owner **Jo Barsky** seemed enthusiastic when I called her later and told her I was thinking of sending bicycle riders past there.

Lunch is served there from 11 a.m. to 3 p.m. Monday through

Saturday. It's all premium food, Barsky said—vegetables fresh out of the garden, hand-pattied hamburgers, freshly made chicken salad, that sort of thing. There are plate lunches.

Dinner is 6 to 9 on Fridays and Saturdays. Saturday there's a hand-sliced Angus prime rib special.

Route Sheet

0.0	Leave Bourbon County Middle School, crossing Paris Pike onto Hume Bedford Road.
5.1	Cross Greenwich Pike.
6.6	Left on Russell Cave Road. Loradale Store.
6.8	Right on Carrick Road
8.9	Home of the great Bluegrass randonneur on right somewhere
9.6	Cross Mt. Horeb Road.
11.0	Left on Stone Road
12.0	Left on KY 922 (Newtown Pike)
12.3	Right on Johnsons Mill Road
13.2	Stay straight on Crumbaugh Road.
14.3	Left on Lemons Mill Road
15.3	Left onto KY 922
15.6	Right onto Lemons Mill Road
17.4	Pass Mt. Horeb on left.
18.2	Left on Old Lemons Mill Road
20.4	Right on Russell Cave Road
20.8	Left on Greenwich Pike (KY 1876)
21.2	Right on Harp Innis Pike
22.2	Follow Harp Innis left.
25.0	Right on Paris Pike (Caution)
25.6	Left on Huston-Antioch Road. Terry's Corner
28.1	Left on Bethlehem Road
32.2	Pass Hutchison Road, stay straight on Bethlehem.
36.6	Back at school

Alternate 1

0.0	Leave Bourbon County Middle School, crossing Paris Pike onto Hume Bedford Road.
5.1	Left on Greenwich Pike
8.8	Left on Harp Innis Pike
9.8	Follow Harp Innis left.
12.6	Right on Paris Pike (Caution)
13.2	Left on Huston-Antioch Road. Terry's Corner
15.7	Left on Bethlehem Road
19.8	Pass Hutchison Road, stay straight on Bethlehem
24.2	Back at school

Alternate 2

0.0	Start at JimTown First Baptist Church, on Jimtown Lane off Greenwich Pike, and go south on Greenwich Pike.
3.6	Right on Russell Cave Road
3.9	Left on Old Lemons Mill Road
6.8	Right on Mt. Horeb Pike
7.1	Straight on Lemons Mill Road
8.3	Left to stay on Lemons Mill
8.6	Right on Lemons Mill
9.8	Right on Crumbaugh Road
11	Right on Johnson's Mill Road
12	Left on Newtown Pike, KY 922
12.1	Right on Stone Road
13.1	Right on Carrick Road
17.3	Left on Russell Cave Road at Loradale
17.5	Right on Hume Bedford Road
19	Right on Greenwich Pike
19.7	Back at Jimtown

Alternate 3

0.0	Start at Jimtown First Baptist Church, on Jimtown Lane off Greenwich Pike, and go south on Greenwich Pike. Right on Greenwich Pike

3.6	Right on Russell Cave Road
3.9	Left on Old Lemons Mill Road
6.8	Right on Mt. Horeb Pike
7.1	Right to stay on Mt. Horeb
9.8	Right on Carrick Road
12.4	Left on Russell Cave Road. Loradale Store.
12.6	Right on Hume Bedford Road
14.2	Right on Greenwich Pike
14.8	Back at Jimtown Lane

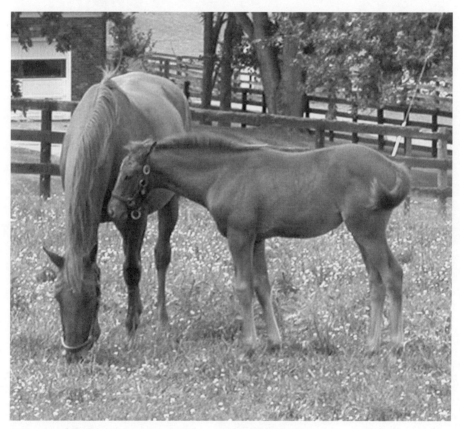

Mare and foal on Mt. Horeb Pike north of Lexington.

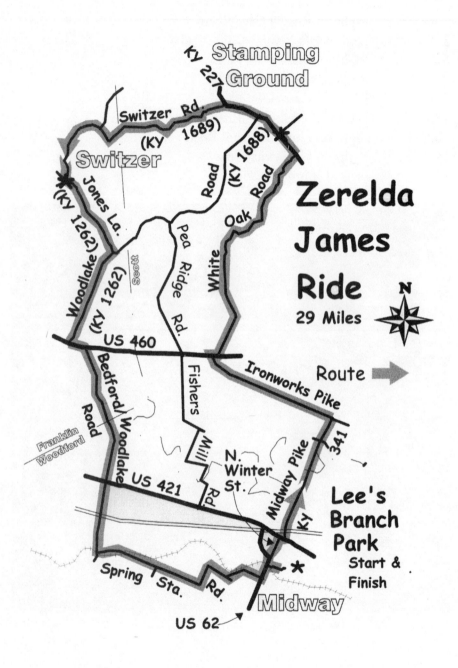

7

Zerelda James Ride

Twenty-nine miles. A bit hilly. Some traffic in Midway and Stamping Ground. Start at Lee's Branch Park at the end of Dudley Street in Midway, Ky. From I-64, about 10 miles west of Lexington, take exit 65. Follow U.S. 62 to Main Street, turn east, jog left on Gratz Street, and take Dudley right to the park.

This is just a nice ride. It gets into the hillier part of the Central Bluegrass, though I avoid some of the big climbs known and loved by riders of the revamped century course added to the Bluegrass Cycling Club's Horsey Hundred ride a few years ago.

It will take you through **Stamping Ground**, which has three main claims to fame as far as I can tell. It was named for the way buffalo had trampled the vegetation all around a spring near the current town when woodsmen first showed up to look it over in 1775. That's one.

Two, **Zerelda Elizabeth Cole** and the **Rev. Robert Sallee James**, who became the parents of **Frank and Jesse James**, were married in Stamping Ground on Dec. 28, 1841. Zerelda was 16 when they married, and attending a convent school in Lexington. And Robert was a Baptist preacher. They moved to **Missouri** a few years later, and Robert died in the gold fields of **California** in 1850.

Zerelda was 5 feet, eight inches tall, and came to weigh more than 200 pounds. She was said to be domineering and outspoken, and very protective of her boys. She lived to be 86, though she lost an arm when **Pinkertons** raided her farm years before that. She died of a heart attack on a train. Which is ironic, because her sons probably gave a lot of people heart attacks on trains.

The Wind It Blew

For the third thing, Stamping Ground was hit hard by one of the tornadoes that swept through Kentucky on April 3, 1974. Reports say the damage was about five miles wide, a record for a tornado. Many buildings were damaged, including the school.

The ride actually starts in nearby Midway, Ky., at Lee's Branch Memorial Park. Make your way out Dudley, Gratz and East Main streets—the latter also known as Railroad Street—and turn right on U.S. 62/North Winter street. U.S. 62 diverges to the left after a bit, but you bear right and then left to stay on North Winter.

U.S. 62 turns to the right in front of you, and you'll rejoin it for just a short distance, to reach KY 341, cross the Interstate, and head out of town. It's all good riding. You'll hit a chunk of Ironworks Pike and cross U.S. 460 to reach the thoroughly delightful White Oak Road. There are no really fancy farms on White Oak, but it's just a joy to ride.

The Long and Winding Trail

Turn left when you reach KY 227, and wheel into downtown Stamping Ground. To me it has a sort of new look about it. Years ago, a rail line that used to run from Forks of Elkhorn, near Frankfort, through **Switzer** and Stamping Ground to Georgetown, was shut down.

There was talk of turning the abandoned roadbed into a long, skinny state park. The idea was quickly scotched by insistence of farmers along the way that the right-of-way should revert to them. But before advocates gave up, I hiked the route with **Al Allen**, then *The Courier-Journal's* photo director, and we did a story about it.

It would have been great. The road was essentially level and the route took you through really rural countryside, across a wooden trestle or two, past the **Switzer Covered Bridge**, and through great places like Stamping Ground. There were a lot of old buildings there then, including a shuttered distillery—the demise of which I gathered was one of the reasons for shutting down the railroad.

Things to Eat

Anyway many of the buildings look newer, including the **Citgo Food and Fuel** on KY 227—or Main Street—almost a mile after you reach 227. You can get good sandwiches and hot food like fried chicken there, as well as cold drinks and snacks. It's open from 6 a.m. to 10 p.m., except on Sunday, when hours are 7 to 9. There's a public rest room.

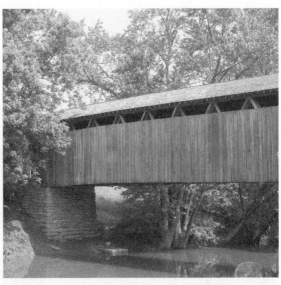

Switzer Covered Bridge, at Switzer north of Frankfort.

If you'd rather have a sit-down dining experience, you can proceed on to **Nancy's Kitchen**, which appears to be in a surviving older building a little bit further down Main Street. **Ann Collins**, daughter of the Nancy whose kitchen it is, describes the cuisine as "home cooking—brown beans, cornbread, chili, fried chicken, things like that." It's open from 5:30 a.m. to 9 p.m. Monday through Friday, and 8:30 a.m. to about 1 a.m. on Saturday, when they have country music in the evening. Closed Sunday.

Waddle On

If you can still get on the bike, take a left on KY 1689 (Switzer Road) a little beyond Nancy's and head down toward Switzer. KY 1689 is a little hilly in spots, but a nice road. Turn left just past the fire station in Switzer and take Jones Lane, or KY 1262. The first thing you see on your left will be the Switzer Covered Bridge, which used to take KY 1262 across **North Elkhorn Creek**. More about that in the Switzer Bridge Ride, next in this book.

Proceed on up a hill or two, and you'll reach a fork where KY 1688 from Stamping Ground comes in to KY 1262. You have to kind of bear right. You cross U.S. 460 with a bit of a jog to the left, and then U.S. 421, and you're back in Woodford County, at **Spring Station**. Take a left and follow Spring Station back into Midway, and back to the start.

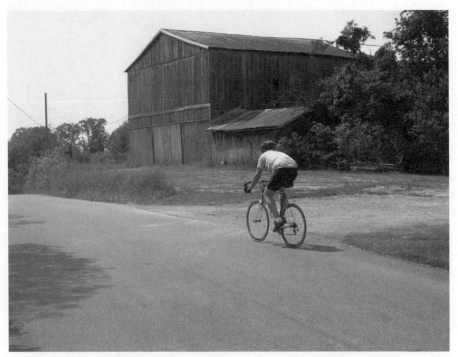

A Horsey Hundred rider tops a hill near a barn east of Switzer.

Route Sheet

0.0	Head out of Lee's Branch Memorial Park on Dudley Street in Midway.
0.3	Left on Gratz, left on E. Main
0.4	Right on U.S. 62 (North Winter)
1.0	Bear right and then left to stay on N. Winter.
1.4	Right on U.S. 62
1.5	Left on KY 341
3.9	Left on Ironworks Pike
6.5	Right on U.S. 460
6.7	Left on White Oak Road
11.0	Left on KY 227
11.8	Pass the Citgo Store in Stamping Ground.
12.7	Left on KY 1689
15.6	Pass Snavely Road, bear left.
17.1	Left on Jones Lane (KY 1262) in Switzer
17.3	Switzer Bridge on left
18.7	Bear right past KY 1688.
20.6	Left on KY 460 for a short distance
20.9	Right on Bedford/Woodlake Road (KY 1685)
23.3	Cross U.S. 421.
24.6	Left on Spring Station Road
28.2	Left on U.S. 62 (S. Winter Street)
28.5	Right on E. Main
28.6	Left on N. Gratz Street, right on Dudley Street
28.9	Back at park

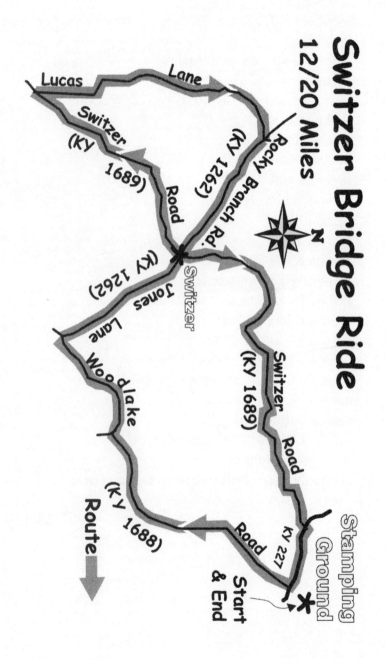

Switzer Bridge Ride
12/20 Miles

8

Switzer Bridge Ride

Twelve or 20 miles. A bit hilly. Moderate traffic. Start on Main Street in Stamping Ground, which is about 23 miles northwest of Lexington. Take I-75 north and use exit 125 on U.S. 460 in Georgetown. Follow 460 to the west edge of Georgetown and then turn right on KY 227. Follow that about 6.3 miles to Stamping Ground.

There's a great covered bridge in Switzer, a few miles out of Frankfort in **Franklin County**, and traditional rides to it have typically gone out of **Forks of Elkhorn**, closer to Frankfort than Stamping Ground, where this ride starts. But it seems to me that traffic around Forks of Elkhorn has picked up in recent years. So I had a look at a couple of routes out of Stamping Ground, and I decided I like them better.

One thing I always liked about riding out of Forks of Elkhorn was Lucas Lane—just a very nice rural highway. So I made a figure eight ride out of this, with Switzer at the waist. Later, when I was looking over my routes to find candidates for shorter rides—as an offering to new riders I hope will buy this book—I noticed that going from Stamping Ground to Switzer on one road and returning on another would make a nice little 12-mile ride—maybe a little hilly, but nothing the rider won't be happy to look back on.

And, if you want a longer ride, either of these routes could easily be combined with the Zerelda James Ride, or even stretched out to include that and the Big Sink Road ride.

Park on the Street

I just parked on Main Street in Stamping Ground. That's along KY

227. There looked to be plenty of spaces to me, and the prospects for returning and finding your vehicle intact seemed good all along there.

What there is to say about Stamping Ground I pretty much covered in the last chapter. It was named for the way buffalo had tramped down all the vegetation around a spring here. Zerelda and Robert James were married here in 1841, and went on to be the parents of Jesse and Frank James. The place almost blew completely away in a tornado in 1974.

Eat Now or Later

But the information on two places to eat probably bears repeating. Both are on Main Street. Citgo Food & Fuel offers good sandwiches and hot food—like fried chicken—as well as cold drinks and snacks. It's open from 6 a.m. to 10 p.m., except on Sunday, when hours are 7 to 9. There's a public rest room.

Nancy's Kitchen, on down the street a ways, offers "home cooking," to include such things as brown beans and cornbread. It's open from 5:30 a.m. to 9 p.m. Monday through Friday, and 8:30 a.m. to about 1 a.m. on Saturday, when they have country music in the evening. Closed Sunday.

Head Down KY 1688

I started the ride by turning off Main Street just a ways past Nancy's, and heading across country on Kentucky 1688, also known as Woodlake Road. It was spring then, and I noticed a lot of blackberry blossoms about 3.5 miles out—something to keep in mind if you happen to be doing the ride in late July or early August.

You turn right when you get to KY 1262, and head on down to the bridge. It seems to me there is a nice downhill there. Remember that for the trip back on KY 1689. But for right now, enjoy this old bridge.

1855 Covered Bridge

The Switzer Bridge was built in 1855 by **George Hockensmith**, who used a Howe truss to reach the 120 feet across North Elkhorn Creek.

Bridge aficionados go for that kind of detail.

It's one of only 13 covered bridges left of 400 that once crossed Kentucky streams. Covered bridges were built at a time when wood was the most readily available material for construction, and all of that elaborate truss-work had to be protected from the elements.

The Switzer bridge held up well until 1905, when its first restoration took place. It carried traffic across North Elkhorn until 1954. Citizens of the area had to fight hard in 1953 to keep highway authorities from tearing the bridge down entirely. They rallied again in 1989 to get another restoration completed by 1991.

The 1997 Flood

Then, in March, 1997, Franklin County got record rains. **The State Journal** in Frankfort reported what happened then from an interview with 14-year-old **Tyler Winn**, whose bedroom overlooked the historic bridge. "There was a cracking sound and I looked out my window and the bridge started moving," he said. "Then it went."

It didn't go far, though. Just downstream is the concrete bridge that now carries KY 1262 across the creek. The covered bridge is bigger. So it got to the new bridge and stopped.

It wasn't easy, or cheap, to get it back to where it came from. It had to be essentially rebuilt, in large part from Douglas fir and Southern pine shipped from **Washington, Oregon and Pennsylvania. Duncan Machinery Movers, Inc.**, of Lexington, which did some of the hauling, estimated that only about 10 per cent of the original bridge remained when the $320,000 project was completed.

One of the Duncan engineers on the job was **Roy Hockensmith**, great-great grandson of George Hockensmith, the original builder.

Moving Right Along

Take a left by the fire station just beyond the bridge, and take KY 1689 down to Lucas Lane—a great road. Back in the early 1980s, **David Runge** and I did an epic three-day camping trip out of Louisville. I was the writer and he the photographer for a Courier-Journal Magazine piece on bicycle camping.

I rode up to Madison, Ind., then crossed over and pedaled to Carrollton, Ky., and camped at **Butler State Park**. Runge joined me the next day, and we pedaled down the exquisite east side of the Kentucky River to Forks of Elkhorn, and camped again. Early the next day we rode out Lucas Lane, and the sun was just so on the large round hay bales in the meadows we passed.

Runge, then a **New Albany High School** art teacher, was beside himself. He kept asking me if I knew about a painter named Monet. It was a memorable morning, and it is the reason I put you today on Lucas Lane.

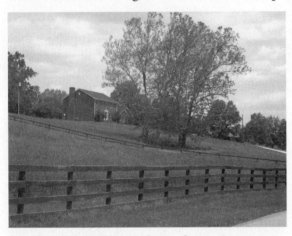

Farmscape on White Oak Road near Stamping Ground.

Close the Hourglass

Lucas takes you up to Rocky Branch Road, and a right that will take you back to Switzer. It's all great riding. Hang a left at the fire station and take Switzer Road, aka KY 1689, back to Stamping Ground. There might be a hill or two in there.

But it's Great.

The Switzer Short Ride

For you newer riders, who want to take in a piece of Bluegrass countryside but don't necessarily want to make an all-day thing of it, I offer the 12-mile version. Just ride down KY 1688 to Switzer, and take KY 1689 back to Stamping Ground. Or vice versa, as they say. In fact, it would be good if you did it both ways, and then got back to me on which is best. I'll put it in the next edition of this book.

Route Sheet

0.0	Leave from Main Street near Citgo station.
0.1	Left on KY 1688
4.7	Right on KY 1262
6.3	Covered Bridge
6.5	Left on KY 1689
9.2	Right on Lucas Lane
13.2	Right on Rocky Branch Road (KY 1262)
14.8	Left on KY 1689
16.3	Bear right to stay on KY 1689.
19.2	Right on KY 227
20.0	Back at start

Short Switzer Bridge Route

0.0	Leave from Main Street near Citgo station.
0.1	Left on KY 1688
4.7	Right on KY 1262
6.3	Covered Bridge
6.5	Right on KY 1689
8.0	Bear right to stay on 1689.
10.9	Right on KY 227
12.0	Back at start

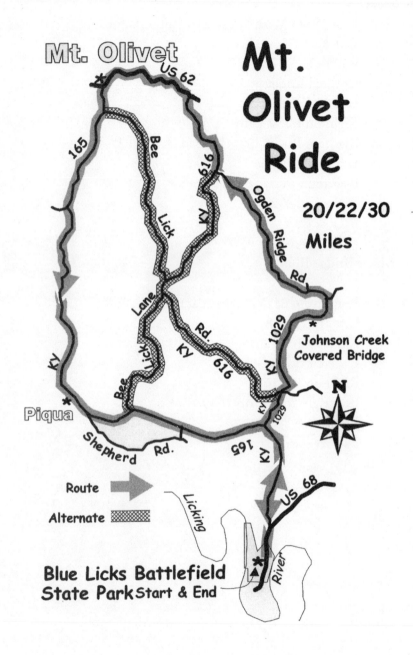

Mt. Olivet

Mt.
Olivet
Ride

20/22/30
Miles

Johnson Creek
Covered Bridge

N

Piqua

Route
Alternate

Blue Licks Battlefield
State Park Start & End

9
Mt. Olivet Ride

Twenty, 22 or 30 miles. A bit hilly, depending on choice of routes. Light traffic. Start at Blue Licks Battlefield State Resort Park, about 38 miles northeast of Lexington, on U.S. 27 and U.S. 68. Take U.S. 27 to Paris, and U.S. 68 from there.

Years ago, when I was a writer in the Courier-Journal's Bluegrass Bureau in Lexington, I was invited to teach journalism at a writers workshop, and one of the other teachers was **Dr. Thomas Clark,** the Kentucky historian. He's always been friendly when I've met him since, so I went down to talk to him about this Bluegrass book. Among other things, I told him I was planning to start a ride or two at **Blue Licks Battlefield State Resort Park.** In that case, he said, I ought to have a look at the country between the park and **Mt. Olivet,** a few miles north. So I did, and he was right.

There are a bunch of ways to ride from Blue Licks to Mt. Olivet and back, and I've mapped out four here. The main one is just about 20 miles long, and goes past the **Johnson Creek Covered Bridge**, and the old Ogden Ridge log school. I've thrown in the others for variety, one in particular for a little longer ride. All of the roads offer some great, sweeping views from ridge tops out across pastures and farmsteads.

My friends David Runge and **Joe Proctor** and I started picking up on the country flavor of the ride just a couple of miles out, when we came on an old barn with a hand-lettered sign urging us to write in **Rooster Mitchell** for jailer. I had noticed some farms down the other side of the battlefield with a lot of individual coops for some fierce-looking chickens. It occurred to our suspicious minds that there could be some cock fighting in the area, and that the candidate for jailer might have at some time been involved.

Head Up US 68

To get started, you can stay at the lodge at Blue Licks park, or just drive up there and leave your car in the parking lot. Head north on U.S. 68. It's not too busy along there, and you won't be on it long anyway. You turn left on KY 165 about half a mile from the park, past the **Blue Lick Grocery**. It's a great grocery, famous in the area for its country ham. We decided to save it for the return trip.

A couple of miles up KY 165 brings you to its intersection with KY 1029, where you take a right past the barn where we saw Rooster Mitchell's sign. A ways farther brings you to a crossroads, where Mt. Pleasant Road goes off to the right, KY 616 climbs back to the left, and KY 1029 continues on down the hill.

1870s Covered Bridge

There's more than one reason to choose the path of least resistance and continue on 1029, which also is called Old Blue Lick Road from that point. A mile and a half or so on down the road you'll see the old **Johnson Creek Covered Bridge** off to the right, where it awaits a reconstruction job locals say has been promised by the state.

Covered bridges are highly revered by some people. They were mostly built in the 1800s, and they involve various kinds of complex trusses and such. In fact, I gather from *The Kentucky Encyclopedia* that the reason covered bridges were covered was to protect all of that early bridge technology from the weather. It was largely made of various kinds of local timber, and rain and snow could do it in.

Aficionados know all about this stuff, and if you show up at a covered bridge, you might run into one. My wife, Suzanne, and I encountered a couple from **Hudson, Ohio,** near **Akron,** who had driven down to see the Johnson Creek bridge and others in the area. **John and Barbara Hanna.** A drug store operator and a teacher. Bridge freaks.

For the Record

For the record, the Johnson Creek Bridge was built about 1870 by **Jacob Bower**, who was well-known in the area for building covered bridges. He used a Smith type 4 truss, which was invented by a **Robert W. Smith** of **Miami County, Ohio**, a couple of counties north of Cincinnati. Smith had a yard in **Toledo, Ohio,** where he cut timbers for bridges, and fitted them together, then shipped them out to locations mostly in Ohio and **Indiana**. Because of that, he has been called the **Henry Ford** of covered bridges.

I don't know if Jacob Bower got the timbers for Johnson Creek from Smith. I do know that his son, **Louis Bower,** came along in 1914 and added iron tensioning rods and wooden arches to the bridge, making it look a little like a Burr Truss bridge. It was closed to traffic in 1966, and got some repairs in 1972, but needs more. It is getting a little cadywampus.

Bob Clements, who owns **Iron Kettle** restaurant in Mt. Olivet and also is chairman of the **Robertson County Tourism Commission**, said the state has been promising for a number of years to restore the bridge. **The Federal Highway Administration Historic Covered Bridge Preservation Program** had, in 2001, proposed an award of $643,432 for the job.

Just to show you how times have changed, Smith used to charge $19.50 a linear foot to build a 120-foot span, siding and roof included. The Johnson Creek bridge would have come in at a slightly lower rate, since it is 110 feet long. But at the expensive rate, it would have cost $2,145 to build.

Climb a Bit

A short distance past the bridge, hang a left onto Ogden Ridge Road. There will be a little climbing, but it's not steep. And what a view. There's a lot of cattle country in **Robertson County**, and you're soon viewing it from a ridge top, looking down on open, green hills that meet each other at every angle. It's the same from KY 616, or from various chunks of Bee Lick Road, and from KY 165, which I chose as a return route.

Amidst the pastures there are picturesque old and new houses, farm buildings and churches. David, Joe and I encountered a field full of donkeys a short ways up KY 616. There's a great looking abandoned church on 616 just after Bee Lick Road departs to the left toward **Cow Hollow**. Bee Lick Road, incidentally has a couple of really big hills on it.

Log School

Ogden Ridge Road feeds into KY 616 as you near Mt. Olivet, and a ways beyond, just before you reach U.S. 62, you'll see an old log building on the left, with renovation underway. That's the old **Ogden Ridge School**, enough of a Robertson County landmark to be on the tourism brochure. Clements said it was in use from 1870 to 1932. Mt. Olivet people are in the process of renovating and stabilizing the structure. They had removed the old floor when David, Joe and I rode by.

A left on U.S. 62 soon takes you to Mt. Olivet itself, a charming small town from its brand new library—with numerous internet-equipped computers—to the old building that once housed the **Louisiana Hotel**, which was host in its day to United States senators, congressmen, governors and other such people.

Mrs. Mayor

We encountered **Nancy Linville** as we rode into town, in front of the **W. T. Kenton House**, where she lives. She was directing some men who were trimming trees. Mrs. Linville is the widow of **Earl Linville**, who was mayor of Mt. Olivet for 35 years.

Her house, an architectural gem with white columns in front, was built by W.T. Kenton, a member of the family of **Simon Kenton**, the noted Kentucky pioneer and friend of **Daniel Boone**. Mt. Olivet also was the home town of **Bill "Boom Boom" Kenton**, a Lexington attorney who served as speaker of the **Kentucky House of Representatives** from 1976 to 1981.

Mrs. Linville is a member of the Robertson County Historical Society, and was eager to tell us about such landmarks as the Robertson County Court House, which was about half finished in 1872 when members of the Fiscal Court discovered they lacked funds to finish the job. Most of the court members were Masons, so the Masonic Lodge decided to put the second floor on the building.

"It is no doubt the only court house in Kentucky which is half-owned by the Free and Accepted Masons," **T. Ross Moore** wrote in his *Echoes from the Century*, published in 1967.

Lynch Law

Moore, who was a Mt. Olivet high school teacher, gathered up information for his 82-page book—a centerpiece for the county's centennial that year—from old newspapers and other records. There are some interesting stories in there.

In 1879, for example, a man named **Richard Molen** left Mt. Olivet without telling anyone where he was going. Townspeople began to become concerned when he wasn't seen or heard from, and especially when an old man named "Boz" Morgan and a couple of his sons showed up in town wearing what appeared to be some of Molen's clothing.

Asked about it, they became confused and couldn't give a convincing answer. Molen had last been seen in the company of the Morgans and some other men, in some woods out on the Bee Lick Road. Ultimately, a brother of Molen's came down from Maysville with a deputy U.S. Marshal, and identified clothing and a valise found at the Morgans' home as his brother's belongings.

The Morgans and several others were arrested, and began giving contradictory answers. It seemed plain to some townspeople that Molen had been murdered, and also clear who had done it. A menacing crowd gathered outside the jail, where "the gleam of polished Derringer and the flash of keen knives bespoke their mad determination," Moore wrote.

A Surprise Ending

Meanwhile, though, a neighbor of the Morgans went poking around the woods where Molen had last been seen, hoping to find some proof of their innocence. He happened on Molen himself, who—it turned out—had left town to find work, but had grown tired of carrying his heavy valise, and had stashed it in the woods. The Morgans, they surmised, had merely found the valise, which happened to contain clothes nicer than their own.

The neighbor got Molen up on his horse and they dashed for town just as the sun was going down, arriving in time to push their way through the mob that had gathered around the jail, and put an end to the proceedings.

"This certainly was a providential deliverance, and should be a lesson to all who believe in and advocate mob law," Moore wrote.

Obtain Food

Nancy Linville recommends **Bob Clements's Iron Kettle** as a place to get lunch, "if you like country food." Joe, David and I can vouch at least for the pie, which is well worth the ride to get it. It's open from 6 a.m. to 7 p.m. Monday through Saturday. On Sundays, it's open from 7 a.m. to 3 p.m. in July, August and September, and 9 a.m. to 3 p.m. the rest of the year.

Around the corner, as U.S. 62 turns and heads out of town, you'll find **Thomas's Grocery**, where you also can get hot and cold sandwiches, soft drinks, snacks and the like. It's open from 7 a.m. to 8 p.m. every day except Sunday, when it's open from 11 a.m. to 6 p.m. Both eating places have public rest rooms.

Mitchell's Store

You also can get a sandwich and snacks, home made pie, soft drinks, and an assortment of crafts, among other things, at **Mitchell's Store**, about four miles down Ky 165 in Piqua. (They say it "pick-way.")

It's a great, old-fashioned store that dates from 1896 and has gone previously by the names **Overby Store** and **Piqua Store. Wendy Mitchell,** the current proprietress, is from New York state.

She visited Piqua when she was in college, with a friend whose grandmother ran the store. She was charmed, and she said, "If your grandmother ever decides to retire and sell the store, let me know."

Years later, the grandmother decided to retire, and the friend called Wendy. She piled everything she owned into a vintage Mustang, and drove to Kentucky and bought the store. That was in the fall of 1994, and she's been struggling to make a go of it since.

She at least has managed to get the store in the **Robertson County**

Tourism Commission's brochure.

The Husband

Oh, and she soon met and married a local man, who was at the store getting ready to head to a job in Maysville when I rode up.

He stuck out his hand. "Rooster Mitchell," he said.

"The write-in candidate for jailer," I said.

"I've got to get those old signs down," he said. The election had been the previous November, and he'd lost. Next time, he said, he'll be on the ballot.

He is not a cock-fighting impresario. He is a registered nurse. His grandmother gave him the nickname when he was a little boy.

Back to the Park

It seems almost like a coast from Piqua back to the park, except for a bit of a climb just before you get back to the Blue Licks store. You could work up an appetite for one of those ham sandwiches—which are good. The store is open from 6 a.m. to 9 p.m., Monday through Friday, and 7 a.m. to 9 p.m., Saturday and Sunday. Other fare includes soft drinks and snacks. There's a public rest room.

And it's just half a mile back to the park from there.

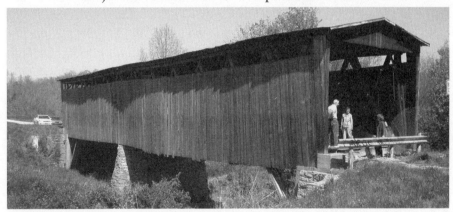

John and Barbara Hanna talk with Suzanne Ward at the Johnson Creek Covered Bridge in Robertson County.

95

Route Sheet

0.0	Leave Blue Licks Battlefield park with a left turn onto U.S. 68.
0.5	Left onto KY 165
2.2	Right onto KY 1029
2.8	Pass KY 616 and Mt. Pleasant Rd. Continue on 1029.
4.3	Johnson Creek Covered Bridge on right
4.7	Left on Ogden Ridge Road
5.0	Pass Old Blue Lick Road on right.
7.6	Right on KY 616
8.9	Left on US 62
10.5	Mt. Olivet. Left on KY 165
14.8	Mitchell's store, at Piqua
18.3	Pass KY 1029.
20.0	Blue Lick Grocery. Right on U.S. 68
20.5	Back at the park.

Alternative one:

0.0	Leave the park with a left turn onto U.S. 68.
0.5	Left onto KY 165
2.2	Right onto KY 1029
2.8	Left on KY 616
8.0	Pass Ogden Ridge Rd.
9.3	Left on US 62
11.5	Mt. Olivet. Left on KY 165
15.9	Mitchell's store at Piqua
19.5	Pass KY 1029
21.1	Blue Lick Grocery. Right on U.S. 68
21.6	Back at the park.

Alternative two:

0.0	Leave the park with a left turn onto U.S. 68.
0.5	Left onto KY 165
2.2	Right onto KY 1029

2.8	Pass KY 616 and Mt. Pleasant Rd. Continue on 1029.
4.3	Johnson Creek Covered Bridge on right
4.7	Left on Ogden Ridge Road
5.0	Pass Old Blue Lick Road on right.
7.6	Left on KY 616
9.8	Right on Bee Lick Road
12.9	Right on KY 165
13.2	Turn around in Mt. Olivet
17.5	Mitchell's Store
20.0	Pass KY 1029
21.8	Blue Lick Grocery. Right on U.S. 68
22.3	Back at the park

Alternative three:

0.0	Leave the park with a left turn onto U.S. 68.
0.5	Left onto KY 165
2.2	Right onto KY 1029
2.8	Pass KY 616 and Mt. Pleasant Rd. Continue on 1029.
4.3	Johnson Creek Covered Bridge on right
4.7	Left on Ogden Ridge Road
5.0	Pass Old Blue Lick Road on right.
7.6	Left on KY 616
12.8	Left on KY 1029
13.4	Right on KY 165
15.5	Right on Bee Lick
17.7	Left on KY 616
17.9	Left on Bee Lick
21.0	Right on KY 165. Turn around in Mt. Olivet.
25.3	Mitchell's Store in Piqua
27.8	Pass KY 1029.
29.6	Blue Lick Grocery. Right on U.S. 68
30.1	Back at park

Blue Licks Battlefield Ride
19/36 Miles

10
Blue Licks Battlefield Ride

Nineteen or 36 miles. Moderate to rather hilly. Some traffic in Carlisle and in places where route takes U.S. 68. Start at Blue Licks Battlefield State Resort Park, about 38 miles northeast of Lexington, on U.S. 27 and U.S. 68. Take U.S. 27 to Paris, and U.S. 68 from there.

I found an article on bicycle touring to The Bluegrass (from Louisville) in an 1896 edition of *The Courier-Journal* that recommended a visit to Blue Licks Springs, about 38 miles northeast of Lexington. The account noted that bloody Indian battles had been fought there, and that, later, it was the site of a famous summer resort to which "The southern planter, in days before the war, came up with a retinue of servants to dawdle away the summer days. . . ."

"Indian arrow-heads may be found in the grim old forest surrounding the springs," it said, and "it is no uncommon thing for a farmer to plow up the bones of some dead brave who fell fighting the paleface, nearly 100 years ago."

Intriguing. Actually, quite a few bones of palefaces ended up in a big grave at Blue Licks, too, and the place figured in a large way in the life of Daniel Boone, over several years.

Blue Licks Springs Battlefield State Resort Park

The state park here, which has had a lodge since 1999, is a good place to start a bike ride. I explored two routes, one up toward Mt. Olivet, Ky.—which is the subject of the chapter just prior to this one—and this

99

one, down through **Carlisle, Ky**. This ride is 36 miles long, and there are a few hills in it, some of them pretty big.

I offer a couple of short cuts, one along Bald Hill Road which can shorten either the main ride or a 19-mile-long alternate by a couple of miles. The trade off is that the short cut is hilly, and a little rough.

The alternate ride skips Carlisle, a thoroughly charming county seat town, and includes a pretty steep hill just off U.S. 68 on Hickory Ridge Road. But both routes are very pretty, and you're riding through countryside that Daniel Boone and other pioneers used to prowl more than 200 years ago.

Daniel Boone and Destiny

The licks are named for the bluish soil to be found around springs that poured out salty water near the bank of the **Licking River**. The salt attracted buffalo in such numbers that they beat out a trail 60 feet wide from the springs to the Ohio River, where Maysville is now. Bones found in the area indicate mastodons and other prehistoric animals trod the same ground before the buffalo.

Boone visited the site in 1774, on a trip to Kentucky to warn surveyors during **Lord Dunmore's War**. He was back in 1776, when he and other settlers from the fort at Boonesborough were on the trail of Indians who had captured his daughter, Jemima, and two Calloway girls from outside the fort. The girls were rescued near here.

Boone was part of a party boiling down water for salt here in 1778 when they were surprised and captured by Indians. Boone spent five months with the Indians, as the adopted son of a chief, but escaped in time to warn Boonesborough of an impending attack by British and Indians, and to help defend the fort in September that year.

And Boone was part of a force from several Bluegrass settlements that blundered into an ambush by British and Indians here in 1782. His son, **Israel**, was among 72 Kentuckians killed.

The White Indian

Simon Girty was a Tory from **Pennsylvania** who had lived with several different tribes of Indians in his teen years, and who threw in with the British during the Revolutionary War. His woods training made him a considerable menace to white settlers all along the frontier during, and for a time after, the war.

In 1782, he cooked up a scheme to use British soldiers and a lot of **Shawnees, Miamis, Mingos, Wyandots, Ottawas,** and other hostile Indians, to lure fighting men out of the Kentucky settlements into an ambush. It worked really well.

The British with a huge host of Indians came down across the **Ohio River** from villages in Ohio, and about half of them hid out around the blue licks. The other half went down and laid siege to **Bryan's Station**, north of Lexington. They let a few couriers through to spread the alarm at nearby settlements, and then abruptly withdrew toward the Licking River.

Listen to Daniel

A sizable force of settlers, led by Boone, **Col. John Todd** and others, had been gathered to rescue the settlers at Bryan's Station, and when they arrived there and found the British and Indians gone, they pushed on in pursuit.

Boone noticed that the Indians didn't seem to be covering their trail very well, and that tracks suggested they were walking in each other's moccasin prints to conceal their numbers. He warned that an ambush was likely. But **Hugh McGary**, of **Harrodsburg**, one of the officers in the group, had been stung earlier by charges of timidity, and he chose Blue Licks to demonstrate his courage.

"All who are not damned cowards, follow me!" he shouted, and charged across the Licking, with the 210 or so Kentuckians right behind. They rode right into 400 or 500 Indians and British, who lay waiting in wooded ravines flanking a bald hill on the other side.

The Battlefield Park

The Blue Licks battle occurred about a year after the British surrendered at **Yorktown**. The word hadn't reached Kentucky. And anyway, the British and Indians kept menacing the Kentucky frontier until the **Battle of Fallen Timbers** in 1794. But Blue Licks is considered the last battle of the Revolution.

A monument to the fallen was erected there about 100 years after the battle, and a state park grew up around it. It's a good place to stay. The food is typical Kentucky State Parks food. Besides the battlefield monument, there's a museum full of pioneer tools and mastodon bones that dates from the 1930s. There is good bike riding all around the park.

Nineteenth Century Hotels

Head out of the park entrance and take a right onto U.S. 68, and another onto Old Maysville Road three tenths of a mile or so later. You'll find yourself rolling through a small community of old buildings, the site of hotels that once drew wealthy patrons from throughout the South.

The Lower Blue Licks Springs Arlington Hotel, which had 300 rooms and was surrounded by verandas, opened in 1845 and burned in 1862. **The Pavilion Hotel**, which had a dining room 100 feet wide and 192 feet long, with a "promenade" all around it was erected later. A **Nicholas County** history says thousands came to the latter resort on Sundays to rent horses to ride and boats to cruise on the river.

The attraction for both hotels was the spring water, said to have medicinal qualities. It also was bottled and sold countrywide for many years. The springs stopped flowing in the late 1890s. Digging intended to find out what happened to the spring turned up the mastodon bones.

Into the Countryside

Old Maysville Road, also named KY 1244 for part of its length, takes you through a couple of right turns south of the Licking River, and then climbs up on a ridge from which you can see cattle grazing on green,

green grass. Keep an eye out for collections of fierce-looking chickens in individual coops on some of the farms you pass.

A couple of miles out you have an opportunity to turn left on Bald Hill Road, which will take you down to **Bartersville**, and save a couple of miles. It is very pretty. But it is hilly, and it gets rough in spots. I chose a loop that takes KY 1244 a bit farther and then cuts across Rose Hill Road, also known as KY 3314, to follow KY1244 once more into Bartersville.

There's a nice little country store a tenth of a mile out on Bald Hill Road, called **D&D Grocery**. You can get snacks, sandwiches and soft drinks there. Part owner **Sheila Garrett** said plumbing problems mean the rest rooms are in operation "sometimes." Hours are 7 a.m. to 7 p.m. Monday through Saturday, and 7 to 5 on Sunday.

Bartersville is also decision time for the main route or the alternate. The former takes KY 1244 on down to U.S. 68, and the latter hits U.S. 68 a bit farther north, by following Mt. Mariah Road, or KY 1455, instead.

Climbing for the Sky

If you take the alternate, you will find Mt. Mariah hilly. And once you cross U.S. 68, you may look up Hickory Ridge Road and say, "Oh no!" You might want to build up a little momentum. Or, it might be a good time for a stroll.

Hickory Ridge takes you around **Lake Carnico**, then up Stony Creek and Blue Licks Spring roads, to a short stretch along the edge of U.S. 68 back across the river and into the park. It does bypass Carlisle, and several stores to be found on the main route.

The main route reaches U.S. 68 near a farm called **Forest Retreat**, which is the site of an ancient stone barn. The place belonged to **Thomas Metcalfe**, a Kentucky governor, congressman and U.S. Senator, who laid the cornerstone for the old governor's mansion in Frankfort.

The farm also is the site of the only known Daniel Boone cabin still in existence in Kentucky. Boone built it in 1795 on land that belonged to one of his sons, and he and **Rebecca** lived there until they gave up on Kentucky and moved to Missouri in 1799. The farm is private, and you can't see the cabin from the road.

Charming Carlisle

A short jaunt down KY 32 takes you into Carlisle, the **Nicholas County Seat,** which has a picturesque court house and a lot of beautiful Victorian houses and buildings. There's a fascinating old graveyard.

As you come into town, KY 32 joins KY 36, and the **Tracks Restaurant** is right there on your right. It has good food at good prices, and if you ask, they'll turn on the electric train that runs on a track around the dining room. It's open from 10 a.m. to 10 p.m. Sunday through Thursday, and 10 to 11 on weekends.

Or, if you don't have time for a sit-down meal, the **Marathon Food Center** next door has snacks and soft

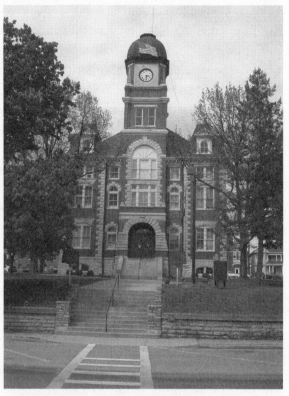

The Nicholas County Courthouse in Carlisle, KY.

drinks, and sandwiches and fried chicken. It's open from 5 a.m. to 10 p.m. Sunday through Thursday, and from 5 to 11 Friday and Saturday. Both have public rest rooms.

Back into the Countryside

Ride right through Carlisle, taking a little time to crank around some of the streets if you like, and take a right turn to stay on KY 36 on the eastern outskirts of town. A couple of left turns put you on scenic Cassidy

Creek Road. That takes you to a short chunk of KY 32, where you will find the **County Grocery and Beer** store.

Owner **David Hardin** said he gets cyclists through there all the time. And they like to sit out on his deck with an Ale-8. The store offers hot food and cold sandwiches, along with the snacks and soft drinks. There's a public rest room. It's open from 7 a.m. to 8 p.m. Sunday through Thursday, and from 6 a.m. to 9 p.m. on Fridays and Saturdays.

Climb a Little, Then Head Home

You follow KY 32 a short distance from the store, and then turn left onto Goose Creek Pike. A short way later, there is a big hill to welcome you onto the pike. After awhile, you will reach the intersection of Goose Creek and Blue Licks Spring Road. But first, Goose Creek will give you another big hill to bid you goodbye for this trip.

A right on Blue Licks Spring Road takes you back to U.S. 68. It used to cross the highway there and take you back to the little Blue Licks community. It still will if you want to walk your bike down a rutted trail in front of an old tobacco barn to reach a narrow stretch of pavement that tends to be littered with tree debris.

Otherwise, just take U.S. 68 on to the park. There may be a bit of traffic, because that road takes people to Maysville, along the same route the buffalo used to take years ago. But the road is nice and wide there, and there's a good shoulder if you need it. Be careful.

Route Sheet

0.0	Blue Licks Battlefield State Park. Right on U.S. 68
0.3	Right on Old Maysville Road
1.4	Right to stay on Old Maysville Road (KY 1244)
2.0	Right to stay on Old Maysville

Note: You can take Bald Hill Road left here, and save about two and a half miles. Bald Hill is pretty, but there are some steep hills, and the road is rough in places.

5.2	Left on Rose Hill Road
6.4	Left to rejoin KY 1244
8.6	Bartersville. Left a tenth of a mile for D & D Store. Otherwise, straight on KY 1244
11.9	Left on U.S. 68. Boone Cabin nearby.
12.1	Right on KY 32
14.2	Join KY 36 in Carlisle, follow it through town.
16.0	Right to stay on KY 36
19.4	Left on Cane Run Road (KY 928)
22.9	Left on Cassidy Creek Road (KY 3315)
27.3	Right on KY 32. County Store
28.1	Left on Goose Creek Pike. Commence big hill shortly.
30.7	Pass KY 1658. Big hill soon
31.9	Right on Blue Licks Spring Road
34.0	Right on U.S. 68
35.8	Back at the park

Blue Licks Alternate

.0	Blue Licks Battlefield State Park. Right on U.S. 68
0.3	Right on Old Maysville Road
1.4	Right to stay on Old Maysville Road (KY 1244)
2.0	Right to stay on Old Maysville

Note: You can take Bald Hill Road left here, and save about two and a half miles. Bald Hill is pretty, but there are some steep hills, and the road is rough in places.

5.2	Left on Rose Hill Road
6.4	Left to rejoin KY 1244
8.6	Bartersville. Left a tenth of a mile for D & D Store. Otherwise bear left onto Mt. Mariah Road (KY 1455).
9.8	Left on U.S. 68
9.9	Right on Hickory Ridge Road. Up a steep hill
11.5	Left to stay on Hickory Ridge, then again almost immediately
12.3	Left on Stony Creek Road
14.2	Right on Blue Licks Spring Road
14.7	Bear left to stay on Blue Licks Spring.
16.8	Right on U.S. 68
18.6	Back at park

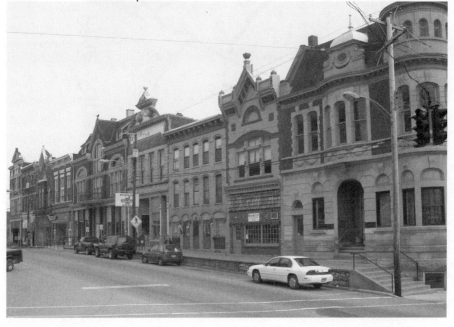

Carlisle, Kentucky

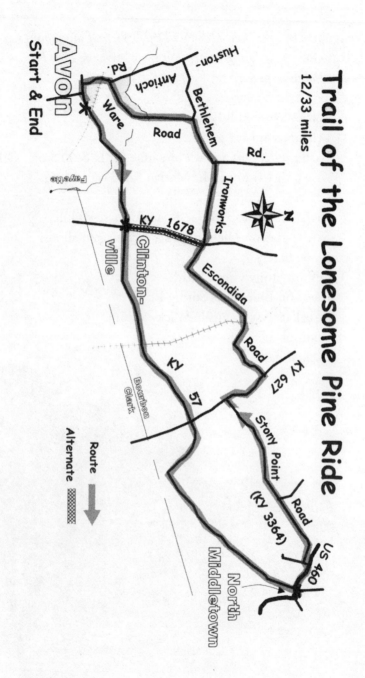

Trail of the Lonesome Pine Ride
12/33 miles

11
Trail of the Lonesome Pine Ride

Twelve or 33 miles. Moderate traffic and hills. Start at Bluegrass Station in Avon, about 12 miles northeast of Lexington. Take I-64 east, and go left off exit 87 on KY 859. Turn right when you reach KY 57, and park near the railroad tracks.

Actually, if there are any lonesome pines on this ride, it is coincidental. The name applies because the birthplace of **John Fox Jr.**, author of *Trail of the Lonesome Pine* and other stories that capture the flavor of Kentucky's Appalachian mountain culture, is about 20 miles out, near Stony Point Road.

Back in 1862, when Fox was born, there was a little town called Stony Point out on this route, and a school called Stony Point Academy, which Fox's father operated. Fox was a precocious child, and he entered Transylvania College in Lexington at age 15. After two years, he moved on to Harvard, where he graduated cum laude in 1883.

He worked on a couple of newspapers in **New York** and served as a foreign correspondent in **Cuba** and in **Mongolia**, but eventually family business speculations moved him to **Big Stone Gap, Va.**, where he stayed to write.

Trail of the Lonesome Pine is about the clash of cultures that occurred when mining interests began encroaching on the mountain culture in Virginia and Kentucky about the time Fox showed up there. Big Stone Gap drew an outdoor drama script from it, which is presented each summer.

Hollywood Calls

Trail got a bit more critical acclaim than Fox's earlier *The Little Shepherd of Kingdom Come*, though both are considered a bit on the melodramatic side by today's standards. *Little Shepherd* was among the first American books to sell more than one million copies, and it was made into a 1961 movie, starring **Jimmie Rodgers**.

It was set in an **Eastern Kentucky** community and was a Civil War tale about a boy torn between his Bluegrass roots and his mountain upbringing.

Fox built an elaborate home in Big Stone Gap based on **Sir Walter Scott's Abbotsford**, and he married an Austrian opera singer who brought a glittering lifestyle to the Virginia mountains. They were divorced after five years, but Fox wrote nothing during their marriage, and little after.

Avon

I offer you here a 33-mile ride, or a 12-mile ride—medium and short. The short ride misses both John Fox's birthplace and **Arthur Hancock's Stone Farm**—to be discussed in a minute—and a lot

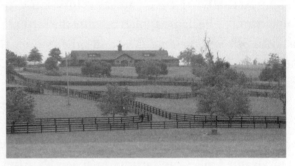

Stone horse barns on Evergreen Farms along Escondida Road east of Paris.

of nice countryside. But it's short, and pretty and nice, if that's perhaps what you're looking for.

Start near the old **Lexington-Bluegrass Army Depot** at **Avon** on KY 57, northeast of Lexington. There always is parking near where the railroad tracks cross KY 57, just east of its intersection with KY 859 which comes over from I-64.

The army facility was a signal depot opened in 1941, and closed in 1995, though the **Kentucky National Guard** still uses space there. The state is in the process of trying to create jobs by leasing light industrial sites in the

110

780-acre complex left behind. But plans also call for a championship soccer complex with up to 20 fields, an outdoor amphitheatre, and an 18-hole golf course to replace the 8-hole course already there.

Store Stops

Ride northeast to Clintonville, at the intersection of KY 57 and KY 1678, and find the **Country Corner Store.** It has sandwiches, cold and grilled, and soft drinks and snacks. There is a public rest room. It's open from 6 a.m. to 8 p.m., except on Sunday, when the hours are 11 to 6. Owner **David Burton** said the grill usually shuts down at 1 or 1:30, but there are always cold sandwiches.

If you're doing the short ride, you turn left here, and then again on Ironworks Pike, almost two miles up Clintonville Road. Then just follow the route sheet back.

If you're doing the main ride, press on here, and enjoy the great countryside up to **North Middletown.** That's about halfway through the ride, and therefore a legitimate place to stop for a snack or a sandwich.

Timothy Morris, proprietor of the **Country Boy Food & Fuel Center,** a bit off the trail to the right on U.S. 460, will be waiting for you. His store makes great sandwiches and has snacks and soft drinks, and offers public rest rooms. There's more about the Rev. Mr. Morris in Chapter 25, the A.D. Ruff Ride, later in this book.

The Country Boy's hours are 6 a.m. to 10 p.m., except Saturday—when they are 7 to 10—and Sunday, when they're 8 to 10.

Arthur Hancock and Sunday Silence

Head back up U.S. 460 toward Lexington, but turn left onto Stony Point Road (KY 3364) a little less than a mile from the store. It will take you over to KY 627 and the John Fox Jr. site. But just before that you'll see Stone Farm on the left.

Three Kentucky Derby winners came from there—**Gato Del Sol,** who won in 1982, **Sunday Silence,** who won in 1989, and **Fusaichi Pegasus,** the 2000 derby winner. It is the farm of **Arthur Hancock III,** son of **A.B.**

"Bull" Hancock Jr., who owned the legendary **Claiborne Farm** on the other side of **Bourbon County**. Arthur III's brother, **Seth Hancock,** now owns the home farm.

Sunday Silence won the Derby and the **Preakness**, and nearly won the Triple Crown, losing the **Belmont** to **Easy Goer**. Sunday Silence and Easy Goer were like **Affirmed** and **Alydar**, or **Nashua** and **Swaps**—always neck and neck in the big races.

Beating Up on Little Brother

But there was an added element of interest between Sunday Silence and Easy Goer. Easy Goer was bred by Claiborne Farm—which Arthur Hancock had left to start his own farm—so there was a sort of sibling rivalry going on. Sunday Silence got the best of it. He was ahead 2-1 after the Belmont, even though Easy Goer had been the prohibitive favorite going into all three races.

And he was the favorite again when the pair met for the last time, for the $3 million **Breeders' Cup** purse in 1989. But Sunday Silence beat him again, by a neck.

Enjoy some more nice countryside on Escondida Road and Ironworks Pike, which is one of the surviving fragments of that old road that carried munitions from iron furnaces up by Owingsville to the Kentucky River at Frankfort during the War of 1812. They were headed for Gen. Andrew Jackson's forces in New Orleans.

Short chunks of Bethlehem and Ware roads, with a little piece of Huston Antioch Road, get you back to the start.

Route Sheet

0.0	Leave Bluegrass Station at Avon on KY57.
3.0	Country Corner Store at Clintonville
6.0	Underpass at Austerlitz
8.0	Cross KY 627
10.5	Pass Pretty Run Road on right.
14.5	Right on U.S. 460 to go to Country Boy Food & Fuel. Head toward Paris on 460 to resume.
15.3	Left on Stony Point Road
19.5	Stone Farm, former home of Sunday Silence
20.0	Right on 627. John Fox Jr. birthplace
21.2	Left on Escondida Road
25.5	Cross Clintonville Road onto Ironworks Pike.
27.4	Left onto 2335 (Bethlehem Road)
28.6	Left on Ware Road, (continuing KY 2335)
31.1	Left on Huston-Antioch
31.8	Left on 57
32.0	Left on 57
32. 5	Back at start

Short Trail

0.0	Leave Bluegrass Station on KY57.
3.0	Country Corner Store at Clintonville. Turn left on Clintonville Road (KY 1678).
4.9	Left on Ironworks Pike
6.8	Left on KY 2335 (Bethlehem Road)
8.0	Left on Ware Road (continuing KY 2335)
10.5	Left on Huston-Antioch Road
11.2	Left on KY 57
11.4	Left to stay on KY 57
11.9	Back at start

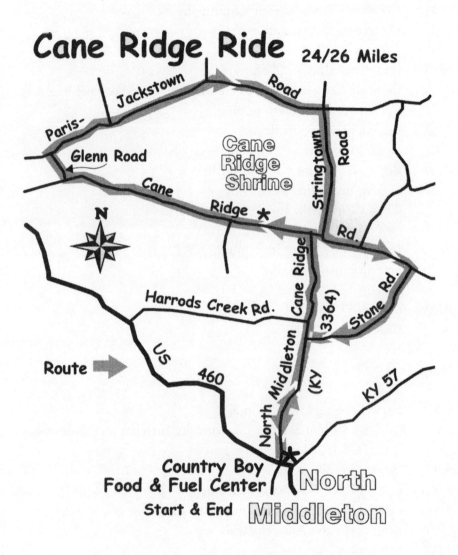

Cane Ridge Ride 24/26 Miles

12
Cane Ridge Ride

Fourteen, 23 or 25 miles. Few hills. Start at Country Boy Food and Fuel Center, North Middletown, Ky., about 26 miles northeast of Lexington. Take U.S. 27 to Paris, U.S. 68 through Paris, and U.S. 460 from Paris to North Middletown.

Cane Ridge Road is a pretty country road that runs out from Paris, Ky., through an area settled around 1790 by people following Daniel Boone's recommendation. Boone reportedly thought it would be rich ground because of the profusion of cane that grew around there. There are a lot of old mansions along the road now, put there—Paris attorney **Roger Michael** told me—by hemp, during that century or more when cannabis sativa was better known for making rope than for smoking.

Soon after the settlers arrived, the Presbyterians among them built a huge log church out there, which was to figure a few years later in a sort of watershed for religion and maybe society in general on the frontier. It is the Old Cane Ridge Meeting House, setting of a famous 1801 revival meeting, a sort of high point in several years of religious revival credited by religion historians with changing the direction of religion in America, giving a big boost to the then-tiny Baptist and Methodist denominations, and generally reducing lawlessness and increasing attention to religion on the raw frontier.

The revival movement actually started a bit earlier in other places in Kentucky, where young preachers far from the seminaries of the east began taking on tones that got their listeners worked up to more than the usual degree. Some in the flock, women at first apparently, started freaking out— shouting and shrieking even, in agony over sins and ecstasy over salvation.

Stoking the Fires

Rather than backing off until decorum returned, some preachers started going with the flow, coming down out of the pulpit and moving through the aisles, stoking the fires instead of cooling them. And people started coming to prayer meetings from miles around.

A young preacher from the Cane Ridge church, **Barton Warren Stone**, who apparently wasn't too convinced that traditional Presbyterianism had a lock on salvation anyway, saw some of that fervor at meetings led by Presbyterian minister **James McGready** in **Logan County**, down on the Tennessee Line.

By the time he called his communion service at Cane Ridge for August 8, 1801, people apparently were really ready. They came from every direction, in wagons and on horseback and afoot, and began converting like there was no tomorrow.

Witnesses wrote later that people, including many women, were laughing and singing uncontrollably, and barking, swooning and running around among the trees in the vicinity of the meeting house. Huge groups collapsed like ripe grain before a big wind, and, while some lay still as death, others twitched and jerked. Sometimes there were five or six preachers going at once, scattered around the grounds on stumps and logs and wagon beds.

Old Time Rock and Roll?

It sounds like a sort of early-day **Woodstock**. To some degree, people must just have let themselves go with the pure joy of being alive and among their fellow humans after a few decades of struggle, loneliness, and danger on a harsh frontier. The birthrate in the area soared nine months later.

Anyway, the old meetinghouse is still out there, encased since 1957 in an outer church of stone. It's in a great setting for the perhaps more subdued but still genuine joy of getting out amidst the trees and fields, under the blue sky, on the saddle of a bicycle.

It is reachable from Paris by U.S. 68, U.S. 460, and KY 537. But those stretches of 68 and 460 have become busy and not much fun to ride on in recent years. So I started this ride at North Middletown, which offers access over less traveled roads.

You have Timothy Morris's permission to park behind his Country Boy Food & Fuel Center on U.S. 460 in Middletown. And that is appropriate, in a way, because Morris is the pastor of a Baptist church in **Hazard, Ky.**, and the Baptist denomination grew phenomenally after the Cane Ridge revival.

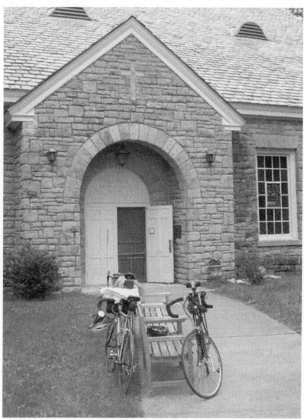

The entrance to the stone building that encloses the 1791 Cane Ridge shrine east of Paris.

The Country Boy's hours are 6 a.m. to 10 p.m., except Saturday—when they are 7 to 10—and Sunday, when they're 8 to 10. There is a public rest room.

Getting the Spirit

I chose a ride that takes you, appropriately enough, north out North Middleton-Cane Ridge Road and then a mile west on Cane Ridge Road to the Meeting House. But that's just five and a half miles, hardly enough to really get into the spirit, as it were, of travel awheel.

So I propose that after you visit the shrine, you continue west on Cane Ridge, take right turns on Glenn and Paris-Jackstown roads, and return to Cane Ridge Road on Stringtown Road.

It's all delightful riding out there, with one whoop-de-do about 15 miles out—just past Blacks Crossroads Road—that could make you get religion. (A whoop-de-do, if I haven't mentioned it previously, is a nice downhill that permits you to get up enough steam to make it almost effortlessly up the uphill that follows immediately. No serious cyclist can avoid feeling a thrill in a good whoop-de-do.)

Endless Options

Back at Cane Ridge Road, you have choice of going left a bit to head back to North Middletown the way you came out, or turning right to add a delightful couple of miles on Stone Road to your itinerary.

So there you have 25.3 and 23.3-mile options. But that's just the beginning. If you wanted to keep it short, you could just ride out to the church and back, for about 11 miles. Or, you could start at the shrine and ride in the other direction, stop at the store for a nice cool Ale-8-One, and return, for the same distance. Or you could take the Stone Road way out— or back, eliminating the Glenn Road loop—making it about 14 miles.

You could just start at the shrine and make the Glenn Road-to-Stringtown Road loop for just over 14 miles. Or, for that matter, this ride— like all those in this book—is readily combinable with others, to make rides of any length. This would combine well with the Avon Depot Ride, for example, or with the Paris-Beth-Paris ride, by taking Ironworks Pike from Bethlehem Road over to Escondida and picking up the Avon route in to North Middletown.

In the last chapter, there is a list of connectors that will get you from any ride in the book to any other ride.

Old Logs

But be sure to save a little of your time to go inside the shrine itself, and absorb the ambience of those two-century-old chestnut logs, which were hacked out of trees when Indian raids from the big villages up in Ohio were still a distinct possibility. It is said to be the largest one-room log building in the country.

There's a gallery, or balcony, built for slaves in the original building that was removed in 1829 as the congregation became abolitionist and the blacks moved downstairs. **Diane Steffer**—co-curator of the shrine, with her husband **Robert Steffer**, when I visited in the spring of 2003—said the gallery spent a bit more than a century as a hayloft in a nearby barn before it was returned in a 1932 restoration.

The shrine is maintained with funding from congregations of the Disciples of Christ, one of the denominations that grew out of that 1801 revival spirit. Groups from several churches use it for services. It is open seasonally, from the beginning of April to the end of October, 9 a.m. to 5 p.m. daily and 1 to 5 on Sunday.

The curators live on the grounds. There also is a museum with a room devoted to church history and a second housing a collection of pioneer tools. It has public rest rooms, and is open when the shrine is open.

Route Sheet

0.0   Leave Country Boy store with a right on U.S. 460
0.2   Right on North Middletown-Cane Ridge Road (KY 3364)
4.7   Left on Cane Ridge Road (KY 537)
5.7   Right into Cane Ridge Shrine. Continue with Right on Cane Ridge Road.
9.7   Right on Glenn Road
10.3 Right on Paris-Jackstown Road
11.7 Pass Tarr Road on left.
13.7 Pass Blacks Crossroads Road on left.
16.2 Right on Stringtown Road.
18.4 Left on Cane Ridge Road (KY 537)
20.4 Right on Stone Road
23.4 Left on North Middletown-Cane Ridge
25.1 Left on U.S. 460
25.3 Back at Country Boy store

Alternate

0.0   Leave Country Boy store with a right on U.S. 460.
0.2   Right on North Middletown-Cane Ridge Road (KY 3364)
4.7   Left on Cane Ridge Road (KY 537)
5.7   Right into Cane Ridge Shrine. Resume with right on Cane Ridge Road.
9.7   Right on Glenn Road
10.3 Right on Paris-Jackstown Road
11.7 Pass Tarr Road on left.
13.7 Pass Blacks Crossroads Road on left.
16.2 Right on Stringtown Road
18.4 Right on KY 537
18.6 Left on North Middletown-Cane Ridge

23.1   Left on U.S. 460

23.3   Back at store

Short Ride

0.0   Leave Cane Ridge shrine, right on Cane Ridge Road (KY 537)

4.0   Right on Glenn Road

4.6   Right on Paris-Jackstown Road

6.0   Pass Tarr Road on left.

8.0   Pass Blacks Crossroads Road on left.

10.5   Right on Stringtown Road

12.7   Left on Cane Ridge Road

13.7   Back at the shrine

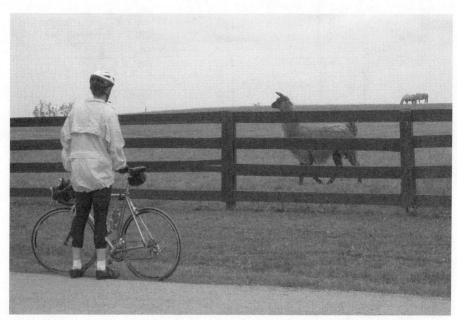

Tom Eblen greets a llama on Stone Road near Cane Ridge shrine.

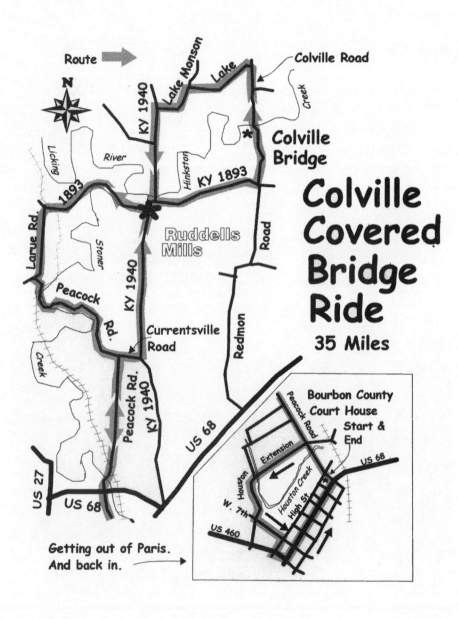

13
Colville Bridge Ride

Thirty miles. Moderate hills and traffic. Start at Bourbon County Court House in Paris, Ky., 15 miles northeast of Lexington. Take U.S. 27 to Paris, and U.S. 68 through town; the court house is on the left toward the north end of town.

This ride is named for the **Colville Covered Bridge** north of Paris, which is an interesting structure. It's 120 feet long and was built in 1887, and you can still ride across **Hinkston Creek** on it. It had to be repaired or rebuilt a few times, to be sure—the last time in 2001. It uses a double post and brace construction, and it used to be a toll bridge. The little white tollhouse is still there. You could cross the bridge free on Sundays, or if you were going to a funeral or to school.

But the real hero of this ride is the little town of **Ruddells Mills,** or maybe **Capt. Isaac Ruddell** himself. Ruddell arrived at the site of the town later named for him, where **Hinkston** and **Stoner** creeks come together to form the South Fork of the Licking River, in 1776. That was during the Revolutionary War, though, and the British and Indians were a menace in those days.

Tense Times at Ruddell's Station

British and Indians laid siege to Boonesborough, about 30 miles almost due south of Ruddells's place, in 1778. They eventually left without taking the fort, but times remained tense in general. In 1779, Ruddell moved his family and some neighbors to a spot almost seven miles down the

123

Licking—almost three miles northwest as the crow flies—where **Capt. John Hinkston** had started to build a fort in 1775.

Things got too hot for Hinkston and his men in 1776, though, and they pulled out. Ruddell and his people made the old fort stronger, hoping to protect themselves against the growing threat. They included 49 fighting men and a couple of hundred women and children and other non-combatants by the time the British showed up in June, 1780.

Capt. Henry Bird, the British commander, had about a thousand fighters, most of them from various Indian tribes, constituting a group that was a bit unruly. Unlike the British forces at Boonesborough, he also had cannon, including a 6-pounder capable of knocking down fort walls.

The Pioneers Lose One

Bird sent Simon Girty—a Pennsylvania Tory known as "the white Indian," who already was infamous among Americans on the frontier—into the fort to tell Ruddell the Indians would probably kill everybody if they had to fight to take the fort. If the fort would surrender, Bird said, the British would take the Americans prisoners, and the Indians would settle for all of their property.

Ruddell reluctantly agreed. But when the gates swung open, the Indians rushed in and began grabbing people as personal captives, separating men from their wives, mothers from their children. They also slaughtered some young, old and otherwise weak people, up to 20 according to some who were there. The dead included an infant torn from the arms of Ruddell's wife, **Elizabeth**, and thrown in a fire.

Those who survived the initial onslaught were marched north, some to the British stronghold at **Detroit,** some to be prisoners in various Indian villages scattered around Ohio.

The Indians, under a different British commander, brought some of the Ruddell's Station captives back to Kentucky 22 months later when they laid siege to Bryan's Station, north of Lexington. Bryan's Station was offered the same surrender-or-die proposition—in a message also delivered by Girty—but the defenders had learned a lesson from Ruddell's Station. They didn't go for it. The British and Indians withdrew, dragging their prisoners back to Ohio.

Years in Captivity

Some of those captured at Ruddell's Station were released in three or four years, as the Revolutionary War ended and prisoners were exchanged. Some had to wait until 1795, after **Mad Anthony Wayne's** victory at the Battle of Fallen Timbers, to head back for Kentucky to find family members from whom they'd been separated 15 years earlier.

Capt. Ruddell and his wife were released with the first group, and returned to their old place at Hinkston and Stoner creeks, where he built a grist mill in 1788, and a sawmill in 1795.

Start at the Court House

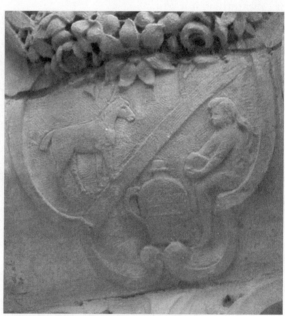

Anyway, there are a few things to think about on this ride. It starts at the north end of Main Street in downtown Paris, at the neo-classical court house, which was finished in 1905. It's considered one of the state's most beautiful, with the four agriculturally-themed murals in its dome.

Stone carving over the door to the Bourbon County Courthouse depicting fast horses, good whisky and beautiful women.

It's worth a little time to wander around. Ask about it. People there are friendly. Over the door to the County Judge's office, for example, there's a big sign that says, "Confederates." I asked why. Nobody knew, not even **County Judge Donnie Ray Foley.** But everybody was happy to talk about it.

"Probably some old confederates put it there," the judge said. **Roger Michael**, a local attorney, took David Runge and me out the door on one end of the court house to show us Kentucky's ideals carved in stone over the door. There was a horse, presumably fast; a woman, presumably beautiful; and a jug of whiskcy.

Down the Hill

Second street takes a sharp downhill right off the bat. I hear some ride leaders in the Bluegrass club like to bring people up that hill, unawares. The first thing I did, though, was find a way around it for the return trip. More about that later. For now, enjoy.

You barely get down the hill when you find Second Street has become Peacock Road, which takes you quickly through some residential areas into the country-side. About three and a half miles out you take a right turn onto Currentsville Road, and soon thereafter a left on KY 1940. That takes you straight out to Ruddells Mills.

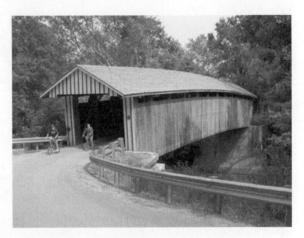

Colville Covered Bridge north of Paris.

There's an interesting store in Ruddells Mills, where you could get a soft drink or maybe a sandwich. Its service seems to be intermittent, though. But we'll be back. So, for the time being, hang a right and go out KY 1893.

The Old Bridge

The Colville Covered Bridge is one of only 13 left in the state, one of only two you can still drive through. It's a mile or so down Colville Road, after a left turn off KY 1893 eight miles into the ride.

126

From there, it's a nice country ride on up to Lake Road, where you turn left, and then bear left where Monson Road takes off to the right a mile or so later. Climb a bit of a hill, and then turn left on KY 1940 to roll back down to Ruddells Mills.

Bluegrass club cyclists occasionally find the Ruddells Mills store open. But not consistently. So take plenty of water. There are no other stores on the route, except in Paris.

Turn right on KY 1893, noting the older houses that befit a place of Ruddells Mills' history, and bear right again to stay on 1893—also known here as Shawhan Road—out toward Shawhan. Cross the tracks and reach Larue Road, then turn left and follow it back to Peacock Road.

1786 House and Martin's Station

You'll cross the tracks there on what looks like a rickety old bridge, though **Lawrence "Lad" Simpson** assured me it is strong. He said there were plans to rebuild it, though. Simpson and his wife, **Pat**, live in that intriguing old stone house on the right after you pass the bridge.

It was built in 1786—just six years after the Ruddell's fort capitulated—by **John Kiser,** a farmer and Bourbon County magistrate. Simpson said a couple of early Bourbon County Fiscal Court meetings, the second and third for that body, to be precise, were held in the house.

Peacock Road continues along Stoner Creek to that intersection with Currentsville Road where you left it awhile ago, and then back into Paris. Somewhere along the creek a few miles upstream from the Kiser house was Martin's Station—a second fort taken by Capt. Bird and his Indians, a day or so after Ruddell's Station fell. They took another 200 or so settlers from there back to Detroit and the Ohio villages.

Simpson said there is nothing left of the old fort on the site.

Hill Avoidance

Now to get you back to the court house without going up that steep hill on Second Street. Head for it, but turn right when you get to the Houston Avenue Extension. That goes around a corner onto Houston Avenue, and reaches 7th Street. Take a left. Take a right at High Street and a left at U.S. 460, and another left on Main Street.

Enjoy those old buildings as you cycle the six blocks or so back to the court house.

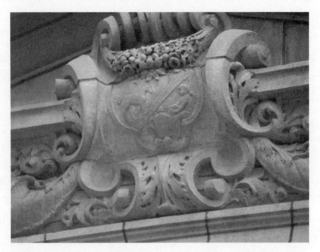

Stone relief at the Bourbon County Courthouse.

Route Sheet

0.0	Leave the Bourbon County Courthouse on Second Street. It becomes Peacock Road. Down the hill
0.9	Cross U.S. 68 Bypass.
3.5	Right on Currentsville Road
4.0	Left on KY 1940
5.9	Right on KY 1893
8.0	Left on Colville Road
9.1	Cross bridge
10.3	Left on Lake Road
11.6	Left at T, still on Lake Road
12.0	Climb a bit of a hill
12.5	Left on KY 1940
13.2	Cross Hinkston Creek in Ruddells Mills and turn right on Shawhan Road, KY 1893.
13.5	Bear right, still on Shawhan.
15.5	Cross tracks.
16.6	Left on Larue Road
19.0	Left at T on Peacock Pike
19.5	Cross tracks on old bridge.
19.6	Old stone Kiser House on right
21.8	Right to stay on Peacock
28.4	Cross bypass.
29.2	Right on Houston Extension
29.5	Left on Houston Ave.
29.6	Left on 7th Street
29.8	Right on High Street
30.0	Left on U.S. 460
30.1	Left on Main Street
30.4	Back at courthouse

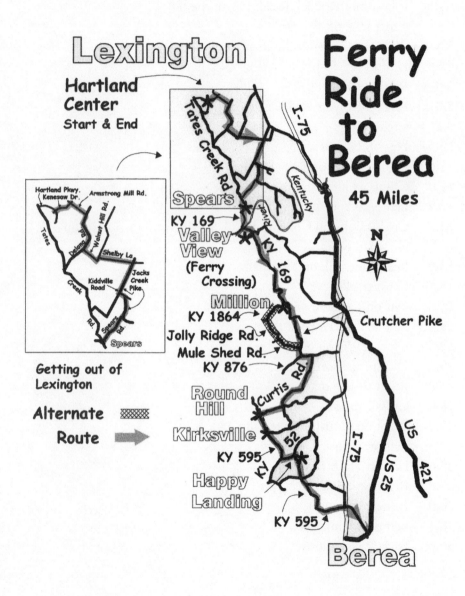

14
Ferry Ride to Berea

Forty-two miles. A few big hills. Light traffic once you clear Lexington, and before you get to Berea. Call ahead - 859-258-3611 - to make sure the Ferry is operating before setting out. Start from the Hartland shopping center, south of Lexington, on Hartland Parkway about three miles out Tate's Creek Road from Lexington's New Circle Road.

When I first started riding bikes with the Bluegrass Wheelmen in Lexington in the mid-1970s, **Dr. Grace Donnelly**, a **University of Kentucky** biologist, was one of the regulars, and—in my case—the one most likely to hang back with a beginning rider and give him or her a pointer or two. I found out recently that she did the same for the now-noted randonneur, Johnny Bertrand, a couple of years later.

She always said riding in the Bluegrass was second only to riding in her native New England, if it didn't exceed even that. Eventually, she went back to New England, and I was sad to learn recently that only a few old-timers in the Lexington club remember her now.

In any case, this was one of her favorite rides, one I told about in a magazine article I wrote on cycling in The Bluegrass in 1976. With some friends, she would head out of Lexington down the Jacks Creek Pike, and take the **Valley View Ferry** across the Kentucky River.

Then she'd pick up the Tates Creek Road in **Madison County** and head on down to Berea, where she would stay at the Boone Tavern and take in one of the arts and crafts fairs, and then pedal home the next day.

Berea and Integration

Berea is an interesting place to go. It's a college town, and **Berea College** has fostered and preserved mountain crafts and mountain culture, which are everywhere in evidence, and give the town a unique flavor. The college recruits poor children, mostly from Appalachia, and charges no tuition. But every student must work a set number of hours in a college industry while in school.

But both town and college were founded before the Civil War to foster racial equality, on land given to the **Rev. John Gregg Fee** by emancipationist Cassius M. Clay. Fee established a church for non-slave holders, and a school. He invited blacks into town to live in neighborhoods with whites.

That didn't fit area mores in those pre-war days, and an armed mob drove Fee and his friends out of town in 1859. They came back after the war.

Fee's college at one time had as many black students as white. The **Kentucky legislature** outlawed such integration in 1904. And though Berea was reintegrated in 1950, that 50-50 ratio has not been achieved again.

The Crafts

Actually, **William Goodell Frost**, who became Berea president in 1892, started moving away from integration as a prime goal of the school, to education of poor whites and preservation of mountain crafts and traditions.

That plan has worked very well. Berea is the acknowledged capital of crafts for Kentucky, and perhaps the region. Craft shops with exquisite wooden musical instruments, all sorts of sculpture and woven goods, pottery and jewelry are everywhere.

In recognition of that unique contribution, the state government opened the $8.75 million **Kentucky Artisan Center** in Berea in July, 2003. The center is expected to draw 400,000 visitors off the I-75 corridor annually.

You've Got Options

I've made this a one way ride, so you could do what Grace Donnelly used to do. Ride down, stay overnight, and ride back. Or, you could make a pretty challenging century of a ride down and back all in the same day.

You also could meet someone for a meal at **Boone Tavern**—which has very good food—or one of Berea's other restaurants, and then let that person haul you home. More about Boone Tavern on the Valley Ride, next chapter in this book.

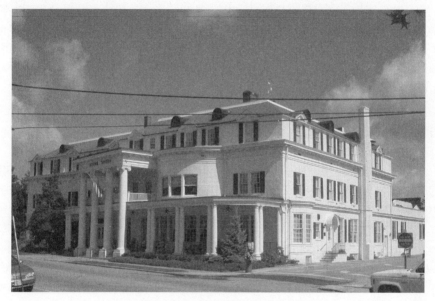

Boone Tavern in Berea

A Creek in Time

You drive out the Tates Creek Road to start this ride at the Hartland shopping center, south of Lexington, in **Fayette County**.

So it may surprise you that you'll be picking up Tates Creek Road again, in the next county, on the other side of the Kentucky River, after your ferry ride. But I've found that to be the case a lot along the Kentucky. Creek roads and ferry roads tend to come in pairs, one on each side of the river.

In this case, according to my map, there actually are two creeks named Tates—or Tate—as well, one on each side of the river. I found a story about the **Madison County** Tates Creek in a book about Daniel Boone, and I suspect it was the first of the two.

When Boone was cutting the **Wilderness Road** from North Carolina to Boonesborough in 1775, he had almost reached his objective when Indians attacked his group in camp near present-day Richmond. A couple of men were killed, and several others narrowly escaped with their lives.

One of the latter was **Samuel Tate**, who got away not by jumping into the canebrakes as everybody else seemed to do in Kentucky in those days, but by running down a nearby creek, thereby hiding his tracks. So they named the creek after him. It enters the river not far from the Valley View Ferry. And another creek by the same name enters the river from the other side in Fayette County, a bit downstream.

Spears Store

There can be a little traffic as you leave the vicinity of the shopping center, depending on the time of day. But it's mostly residential and ordinarily not too high speed. The Bluegrass club has rides from the center regularly.

There are a lot of turns early in the going, and different street names, so follow the route sheet carefully. Soon you should find yourself at the **Old Country Store** in **Spears**, and the route is pretty straightforward from there.

The store, a delicatessen with a full line of sandwiches and tables on the porch so you can enjoy them al fresco, is a pretty interesting place itself. **Tony Konkler**, son of the owners, said it's at least 100 years old, and has gone by many names. "Whoever Owned it Grocery," he said.

And it's a store with a past in every sense of the word. "This was Little Chicago back in the '20s," Konkler said. "If you wanted to get bootleg whiskey, a woman, whatever, you could get it here."

The store is open from 6 a.m. to 6 p.m. daily, and from 9 to "3 or 4" on Sundays. There's a public rest room.

Rollin' on the River

Spears also has **Woodie's Market,** across Tates Creek Road and down a bit from Konklers' store. It has snacks and soft drinks, and is open from 6 a.m. to 7 p.m. Monday through Friday, from 7 to 7 on Saturday, and 7:30 to 6 on Sunday.

From there, you've got essentially a two-mile coast down to the ferry at Valley View. Be careful.

You're about to be a customer of the oldest recorded business in Kentucky. The Virginia legislature gave **John Craig,** a revolutionary war hero a "perpetual and irrevocable franchise" to operate a ferry at this particular point in 1785, and it's been in operation ever since—except during times of really high water.

Seven different families have owned it, including Craig's, but in recent years the counties of Fayette, **Jessamine** and Madison have operated it through the **Valley View Ferry Authority.** So it's free—sort of an extension

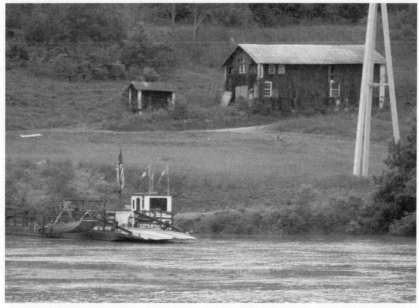

This ferry, on the Kentucky river south of Lexington, has been in operation since 1785, and is the oldest continuously operating business in Kentucky.

of the road.

And if you're worried about going out on a significant river on a 200-year-old boat, don't be. The boat—now called the *John Craig*—was rebuilt except for the paddlewheel and engine in 1996, and the guide wires were replaced in 1998.

Schedule

The ferry ordinarily operates from 6 a.m. to 8 p.m. weekdays, 8 to 8 on Saturday, and 9 to 8 on Sunday. But it is subject to breakdowns, inspections, floods, and winter shutdown. So it's a good idea to call (859-258-3611, and choose option 2) to make sure it's operating before you pedal down the hill.

And speaking of that, you'll be climbing out of the river valley again once you disembark on the Madison County shore, after a look around at the old town of Valley View. They say that many years ago it was bigger than Lexington. It is intriguing.

The hill doesn't really seem that bad to me. And five miles up the road, you'll come to the **Little Ferry Market**, an excuse to stop. They have cold drinks and luncheon specials there, such as beans and cornbread on Wednesdays, and an open face roast beef sandwich on Fridays.

Donna Bailey had been running the store for about a year in 2003. There are rest rooms, "for customers."

The Crutcher Pike Question

Seven miles from the ferry, you'll come to the crossroads town of **Million**, where you have to decide how rustic you want this ride to be. Straight ahead is Crutcher Pike, which can be a little rough, and has a steep hill on it. Some Bluegrass riders prefer to turn left and go around Crutcher Pike by taking KY 1864, Jolly Ridge Road, and Mule Shed Road, a route that adds about two miles to the route. And goes up a different big hill.

When my friend, David Runge, and I were checking this route out, it was early spring and there was some debris on Crutcher Pike. The pavement was crumbled in places. Runge loved it. He is famous in the Louisville Club

136

for "Runge Roads," which tend to be in out of the way places, and sometimes not too recently paved, but always scenic.

We noticed Dan Henry arrows—traditional cyclist roadway paintings—suggesting that the Lexington club had used the KY 1864 alternative at least some of the time. So we checked it out, too. It's very nice, though there is that hill.

Despite the great road names on the alternate route, I think I'd go up Crutcher. But you've been warned that the question does arise.

Boondocks

If you didn't adequately fortify yourself with soft drinks or **Gatorade** at Donna Bailey's place, you'll get another chance at the **Wilgreen Lake Marina,** half a mile off the route about seven miles past Million.

The marina is open from daylight to dark. It has snacks and soft drinks, and no public rest room. But it has plenty of live bait.

Winkler's General Store, also called **Round Hill Store** is a couple of miles further along at the end of Curtis Pike. It has snacks, soft drinks and sandwiches, and a public rest room. Doug Tussey is the proprietor. It is open from 7 a.m. to 8 p.m. seven days a week.

You'll get on KY 595 at **Round Hill**, and it will take you down to **Kirksville**, where you join the **Adventure Cycling Association's TransAmerica Trail**, a bicycle travel route that stretches from Oregon to Virginia. It looks just like any other series of country roads. But you might encounter some cross-country cyclists along here. They almost always have good stories.

On Down to Berea

From Kirksville, you stay on KY 595, though it follows KY 52 for a short stretch. Take it right down under I-75 and into the heart of Berea - right to the doorstep of Boone Tavern, in fact. More about that in the Valley Ride, next chapter.

Route Sheet

0.0	Straight on Kenesaw Drive
0.7	Right on Armstrong Mill Road
1.6	Right on Delong Road
3.4	Left on Walnut Hill Road
4.4	Right on Shelby Lane
6.1	Right on Jacks Creek Pike
7.7	Left to stay on Jacks Creek Pike
8.0	Bear right to stay on Jacks Creek. Kiddville Road goes straight.
9.0	Bear right to stay with Spears Road (KY 1975). KY 1976 goes to left.
9.8	Join Tates Creek Road in Spears. The Old Country Store. Also Woodie's Market.
11.8	Valley View Ferry. Cross the river, then ride straight on KY 169.
14.1	Pass through Stringtown.
16.2	Little Ferry Market
18.0	Million. KY 1984 goes right.
19.3	Straight on Crutcher Pike. A bit of a hill.
21.4	Mule Shed Lane comes in from the right. Name changes to Mule Shed.
23.1	Left on KY 876
23.8	Right on Curtis Road
25.7	Pass road to Wilgreen Lake boat ramp (half mile left).
28.0	Right to stay on Curtis Pike (Winklers General Store)
29.6	Left in Round Hill, onto KY 595
30.8	Cross KY 1295 in Kirksville. Continue on Ky 595. Note beautiful church.
32.8	Left onto KY 52 East
33.6	Right onto KY 595 South, in Happy Landing.
39.6	Cross I-75.
42.0	Boone Tavern

Alternate takes KY 1864 west from Million, and follows Jolly Ridge Road, and Mule Shed Road to get around Crutcher Pike. It adds about two miles to the route.

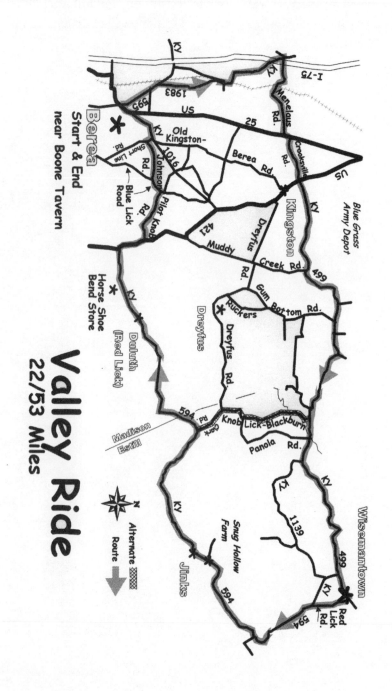

Valley Ride
22/53 Miles

15
The Valley Ride

Twenty-two or 52 miles. Moderate hills and traffic. Start near Boone Tavern, at the intersection of U.S. 25 and KY 595 in Berea, Ky. It's about 38 miles south of Lexington on I-75.

In the early part of the last century, Berea College President William Goodell Frost and Berea professors used to go into the mountains of Eastern Kentucky looking for folk crafts and folk lore, which they hoped to understand and preserve, and teach at the college. They were very successful.

They would invite mountain people to come down to the college and bring their dulcimers and baskets and weavings and talk about them to students, and demonstrate how they were done. Such people were guests of the president, and they'd stay at the president's house.

Nellie Frost, the president's wife, was a good sport about it until one summer the number of guests reached 600. She suggested the college needed a guest house that would give everybody more room. So the College built Boone Tavern, and staffed it largely with student workers, as it does with most college enterprises.

Not to be Confused with Duffy's

Boone Tavern is a tavern in the sense of a waystation where a weary traveler could stop for a bite to eat and a warm bed before continuing on his way. It was named that because Berea is on **Boone's Trace**, the road Daniel Boone built from North Carolina to Fort Boonesborough, which is a bit

141

north of town, in 1775. It doesn't serve liquor.

In fact, until 1999, you couldn't get into the dining room at Boone Tavern without a coat and tie. **Sam McConnell**, guest services manager, told me the hotel began getting many tour groups that came through town on buses, for whom it was hard to pack jackets. They couldn't let them starve, so they relented on a rule strictly enforced by **Richard Hougen**, who was the tavern's chef for many years.

The dining room became famous for Hougen's delicacies, including spoon bread, a sort of corn bread soufflé that it is hard to get enough of. It's a good place to eat, even if you don't stay at the hotel.

Hand-Crafted Rooms

But you should give consideration to staying at the hotel. It has 58 rooms, furnished with fine hand weavings and other crafts made in the college's craft programs. There's a gift shop that offers beautiful crafts—wood carvings, metal sculpture, textiles—made by students.

The tavern serves as a starting point for tours of **Berea College**, a unique school that focuses on mountain crafts and culture, recruits many of its students from mountain poor, and puts all students to work to earn part of their way. The tours, led by students, are offered at 9 and 10 a.m. and 1 and 3 p.m. Monday through Friday and at 9 and 2 p.m. on Saturday.

Ride your Bicycle

I was obviously quite taken with Berea and Boone Tavern, but my original purpose in going there was to check out a ride first suggested to me by Thomas D. Clark, the Kentucky historian, who owns some land along Red Lick Road, and thinks it is beautiful country.

He's right. I found out the Bluegrass Cycling Club has been doing various versions of what noted cyclist Bill Fortune calls "The Valley Ride," with reference to the Valley of Red Lick Creek, which is what Clark had told me about.

It was along Red Lick Creek, Clark said, right where the road makes a near circle to get around Haystack Mountain a little southwest of **West**

Irvine, Ky., that Daniel Boone camped with **John Finley** and others in 1769 and got his first real taste of Kentucky.

Finley had traded with Indians in Clark County northwest of that campsite years earlier, and had told Boone about the wondrous land to be had in Kentucky when they were both wagoners in the French and Indian War. Finley finally searched Boone out in North Carolina and talked him into a foray west of the mountains.

That camp, which was in a clump of trees off the left side of the road as you go around the mountain, was, in a sense, the cradle of U.S. civilization beyond the seaboard. Think about that as you go by.

First, You Have to Get out of Berea

I started this ride right at Boone Tavern because I was so taken with Berea, and Boone Tavern is the heart of Berea. But you can start anywhere in that vicinity. Head out KY 595 past the innovative and singular-looking **Berea Community School** complex on the left, and turn right on KY 1983.

You work your way up to a crossing of Interstate 75, and then across Menelaus and Crooksville roads to KY 499. After that, it's all one road all of the way to **Wisemantown**. And a great road it is. As you get farther east you begin to see the mountains poking up here and there, and, to your delight, hardly climbing at all.

There are a number of communities along the route, none of which seem to have stores any more, but most of which have churches. You will ride along the edge of the Blue Grass Army Depot, which gets in the news every once in awhile because of the nerve gas stored there. But don't worry, it's in steel-reinforced concrete igloos covered by several feet of earth, and locked up inside security like that at Fort Knox.

Food in West Irvine

There ought to be a store in Wisemantown, and until recently there was one. The building it occupied is still there, but it has become a sort of second-hand shop. To get soft drinks and the like, you have to stay on KY

499 to its intersection with KY 52, in West Irvine. There are restaurants there, such as McDonalds, and a place called Cedar Village, where you can get fried green tomatoes, among other things.

If you need provender, you have to add four miles to the trip, because it's two into West Irvine, and two back to Red Lick Road, which we're going to take south from Wisemantown.

In the distance, you'll see the aforementioned Haystack Mountain, which will loom large, and you won't see how you're going to avoid some climbing. But the road just goes around it. It's amazing. You climb a little on the far side, but nothing like you have expected. Don't forget to look on the left for a clump of trees that might have been Daniel Boone's camp.

Wilson Cemetery

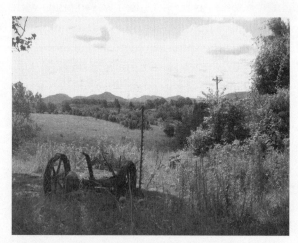

As you pedal east on KY 499 from Berea, the mountains rise in the distance.

A bit before you get to Haystack Mountain, watch on your right for Wilson Cemetery Road. **Captain John Wilson**, of the Federal 8th Kentucky Infantry in the Civil War, is buried there. He and five other Estill County soldiers planted the Union flag at the top of Lookout Mountain in Tennessee, during the battle of that name, in 1863. Wilson lived until 1896 and they buried him there. I didn't go look at the grave, but you might.

Snug Hollow Farm, B & B

After you round Haystack Mountain and head back west on KY 594, you will come to McSwane Branch Road, on the right, which is the address of **Snug Hollow Farm**, a bed and breakfast you might want to give some thought to.

It is operated by **Barbara Napier** and her crew in a three-story house she built over a period of years while living in an old log cabin, which is now being restored as well for guest quarters.

You won't be able to see the place from KY 594, because it's a mile and a half up a gravel road. But Barbara, who cooks all vegetarian dinners on a big old wood cook stove, likes bicyclists and has them as guests often. She will haul you into and out of the farm if you'd like to stay there.

Anybody who has been around any part of the mountains very long will recognize Napier as a good mountain name. And Barbara promises you'll get a good taste of mountain culture at her place, without air conditioning, without television, but with lots of books and with trees and mountains around. Her number is 859-723-4786.

Options. You've Got Options

You could do the main Valley Ride from there instead of Berea, if you wanted to. Or, you could do a shorter, 22-mile version by cutting up Clark Road a little past the B & B and then Knob Lick-Blackburn Road up to KY 499 at Panola. Then you'd just follow KY 499 to Wisemantown and Red Lick Road the rest of the way around.

If you didn't want to stay at Snug Hollow Farm, you could do the shorter version of the ride by parking at the shopping center on KY 52 in West Irvine. (You also could do the main ride from the West Irvine end.)

Horse Shoe Bend

On down KY 594 past Snug Hollow and past the picturesque village of Jinks, KY., you will finally come to a country store on the route. **Horse Shoe Bend**. It's not one of those good old stores that have been around in the same building for years and years, because it burned down a few years ago.

People in the community got together and put it back up. There's a copper plaque on the wall by the door listing the people who helped and thanking them. The owners are **Bonita and Brian Isaccs**, and their son, **Russell Isaacs**, and his wife, **Brandy Isaacs.**

It's a grocery with hot and cold sandwiches from a deli counter. Soft drinks, snacks, live bait. It's all there. Public rest rooms, too. It's open Monday through Friday from 6 a.m. to 9 p.m., Saturday from 7 to 9, and Sunday from 9 to 6.

From there it's not far back to Berea. You will have to take a short stretch of U.S. 421, which can be busy. But you're not on it long. You turn left on Pilot Knob Road, and the knob itself will be very evident. It's not the **Pilot Knob** from which Daniel Boone first saw the Bluegrass, though.

That's up in Powell County. Another ride for another day, and book.

Route Sheet

0.0	Leave Boone Tavern on KY 595.
1.2	Right on KY 1983
4.6	Left on Caleast Road
5.4	Cross I-75 and turn right on Caleast Road.
6.0	Right on Menelaus Road. A little rough at first.
9.0	Left on U.S. 25
9.3	Cross bridge and turn right on Crooksville Road, KY 499.
10.7	Jog left, then right across U.S. 421.
13.8	Pass Muddy Creek Road on the left.
15.6	Pass KY 374 at Speedwell.
16.2	Pass Gum Bottom Road on the left.
17.2	Right on KY 499 at Brassfield. Brassfield Road goes left.
19.3	Left on KY 499 at Panola. Walter Lakes Road goes right.
20.3	Pass Panola Road on left.
22.3	Big hill
25.3	Pass KY 594.
26.1	Wisemantown. Add four miles if you go in to KY 52 for food. Left turn on Red Lick Road (KY 3328)
27.1	Pretty good hill. Stay straight to join KY 594.
30.1	Go around Haystack Mountain, then climb a little.
32.7	Jinks, Ky.

37.4	Bear left on KY 594.
43.3	Horse Shoe Bend Store
46.1	Right on U.S. 421
47.0	Left on Pilot Knob Road (Notice the knob on the left.)
48.7	Left on Blue Lick Road
49.2	Straight on Johnson Road
50.5	Right on Short Line Road
50.7	Left on KY 1016
51.9	Left on U.S. 25
52.3	Back at Boone Tavern

Alternate: If you start the ride at Snug Hollow Farm, you could leave the route from KY 594 at mile 37.4 and take Clark Road and then Knob Lick-Blackburn Road up to KY 499 at Panola. Then follow KY 499 and Red Lick Road back to the B&B, and you'll have about a 22 mile ride. Another starting place would be one of the parking lots in West Irvine, where KY 499 reaches KY 52. Add four miles if you do that.

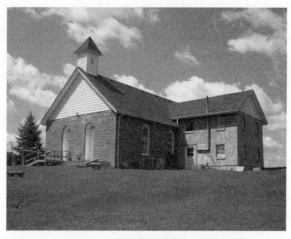

This old church is on KY 499 east of Berea.

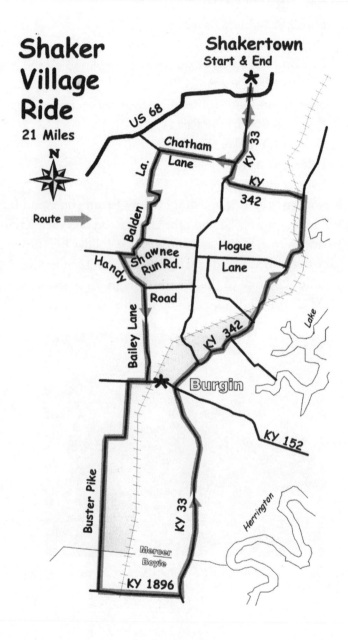

16
Shaker Village Ride

Twenty-one Miles. One significant hill. Some traffic on KY 33.
Start at Shaker Village at Pleasant Hill, 23 miles south of
Lexington on U.S. 68, or 40 miles south of Frankfort on U.S. 127
and U.S. 68 (with a left turn at Harrodsburg.)

The one place I know of where you can see the Bluegrass as Daniel Boone and **James Harrod** saw it—as a savanna-type prairie with a patchwork of deciduous forest and some canebrakes around—is on the restored prairie land of the **Shaker Village at Pleasant Hill.**

Shaker Village, or Shakertown, as most people call it, is really a remarkable place in many ways. The Shakers were a religious sect that peaked in the first half of the 19th Century, at Pleasant Hill and several similar communities around the country.

They may be best known now for their belief in celibacy, one of the factors that led to their near extinction, and for their withdrawal from the outside world. But in their time, they were known for the quality of the goods they produced—a value that lingers in the simple beauty of the buildings and furnishings in the restored village.

The Shakers at Pleasant Hill flourished in agrarian times before the Civil War, working their fertile land to feed and clothe their own 500 members, and also shipping vast quantities of goods to the "world's people." They had big warehouses down the steep, rocky wagon trail from the village to the Kentucky River.

From those buildings, they loaded exquisitely-made goods— brooms, bonnets, pincushions, willow baskets, cloth, herbs, seeds, cloaks,

149

oval wooden boxes, weaving implements, shoes, butter, cheese, livestock and meats, among other things. It all went out on flatboats at first—then steamboats—and was shipped as far downriver as New Orleans.

An Early Day Extension Service

Though the Shakers lived to themselves, they very much participated in the agricultural world of their day, experimenting with plants and animals and developing successful varieties that helped make their neighbors prosper as well. They also put ingenuity into labor-saving devices, and invented the flat corn straw broom, the wooden clothes pin, the circular saw, and a commercial-size washing machine.

There were some chinks in their armor, though. They survived by recruiting new members in an era when religious fervor and revivalism were widespread. That spirit waned in the general population as the 19th century progressed, and they weren't able to recruit dependable adults at Pleasant Hill after about 1845.

Northern and Southern armies advanced and retreated over their land during the Civil War, appropriating their livestock and vehicles, and drawing heavily on their food supplies. They never recovered from that. The war also interfered with their markets downriver. And their craftsmanship could not compete with the mass production that came with industrialization after the war.

So they dwindled in number and went out of business in 1910, and the last Pleasant Hill member died in 1923.

Second Coming

The restoration of Shaker Village, which commenced in 1961, is maybe the second most remarkable thing that has happened on that pleasant knoll above the Kentucky. The Shakers had turned what was left of their 4,500 acres and 270 buildings over to a Harrodsburg merchant in 1910 in return for his care of the last Shakers, and he auctioned the property in 1924.

Many of the buildings disappeared, but the large main ones were built so well that they survived a succession of owners and uses—including a restaurant, stores, service stations, a Baptist Church, tenant housing—in what became a secular, unincorporated rural community called Shakertown, astride busy U.S. 68.

Preservation-minded Kentuckians got together in 1961 to plan a way to restore the village, and hit on the idea of converting it into a sort of museum-resort-farm that would both preserve something of the Shaker culture, and be largely self-supporting.

They managed to hire **James Lowry Cogar**, who had been the first curator of **Colonial Williamsburg** in Virginia, and who happened to be a Kentucky native, to oversee the work. He insisted on buying 2,250 acres of the original shaker land, to serve as a buffer against development—a move that seems ever more prescient as time goes on.

The Magic of Simplicity

So now there is a place you can go to eat great southern food, to stay overnight in 19th century dwellings—with modern amenities—to hike, see costumed presenters demonstrate Shaker skills, take riverboat rides, or learn how to make boxes, baskets or rocking chairs. You can hear the haunting tones of Shaker music and learn how Shakers lived.

"For a week or a weekend," village literature says, "Shaker Village offers you a chance to discover the magic of simplicity."

It sounded like a great place to start a bike ride to me. So I scouted out a couple of routes, with the help of village officials and from David Runge—chief scout for the Bike Trek to Shakertown, a three-day fund-raising bicycle event put on by the **Kentucky Lung Association** that centers on the village each September.

The "lungers" ride all of the roads around Shakertown and through the countryside east and west. It's good riding.

Jacob Froman Farm

Just for a taste, leaving you some time to explore some of Shakertown's offerings, I'm sending you down KY 33 for this 21-miler. There's a bit of a hill on Chatham Lane, right near the start, and a chunk of

KY 33 coming back from KY 1896 can be a little busy, depending on time of day.

Otherwise, nothing should interfere with your enjoyment. You get a good look at the countryside from which the Shakers drew their first Kentucky recruits, though it is changed now by encroaching residential areas and traffic connected with nearby **Herrington Lake**.

Going down Handy Pike, you will pass a section of the huge **Anderson Circle Farm** that is the site of the Jacob Froman house, which dates to 1785 and may be the oldest standing residence in Kentucky. (Read more about Anderson Circle Farm in the New Providence Church Ride, next chapter.)

Ralph Anderson, a very preservation-minded person, acquired the house with some farmland he wanted, and was thinking about tearing it down when he discovered logs under the plaster on an interior wall. Turned out there was a whole log house under the clapboards. His researches traced it to Froman, and the possibility that it is historic indeed.

The property also includes an old barn Anderson thinks may have been built by Shakers. They are studying it.

Burgin

You'll go a couple of times through Burgin, which was an important crossroads town for defense travel between **Ft. Harrod** and nearby outposts in the earliest days of settlement. Burgin is on the Adventure Cycling Association's TransAmerica Trail, a bicycle route initially developed from the country's bicentennial celebration, that runs from Oregon to Virginia.

You might encounter a cross-country cyclist there, most likely at **The Trading Post**, just off KY 152 on the Shakertown Road—where you can get sandwiches, snacks and soft drinks, and use a public rest room. It's open from 5:30 a.m. to 10 p.m. daily, except Sunday, when it doesn't open until 6:30 a.m.

First, Though, the Rest of the Ride

You'll pass The Trading Post on your way back toward Shakertown, after enjoying a ride down Buster Pike to a left turn at the impressive complex of **Immanuel Baptist Church** on Kentucky 1836. Then zip back up KY 33, watching the traffic along there. A little after you pass through Burgin the second time, you'll veer off KY 33 to KY 342, which is a bit less busy.

That will give you a close up look at **Kentucky Utilities Co.'s E.W. Brown Generating Plant**. Depending on the time of year, there are falcons nesting on those stacks.

Then rejoin KY 33, pick up the view of Shakertown's majestic stone fences, and zip across U.S. 68 to leave the 21st century behind.

Route Sheet

0.0	Leave parking lot at Shakertown, cross U.S. 68.
1.0	Right on Chatham Lane. Hill.
2.2	Left on Balden Lane
3.7	Right on Shawnee Run Road
4.3	Left on Handy Road
4.9	Right on Bailey Lane
6.4	Right on KY 152
6.8	Left on Buster Pike
10.3	Left on KY 1896 at Immanuel Church
11.6	Left on KY 33
14.2	Cross KY 152.
14.8	Right on Curdsville Road (KY 342)
17.8	Left on KY 342 E.W. Brown Generating Station on right
19.3	Right on KY 33
20.6	Back at start

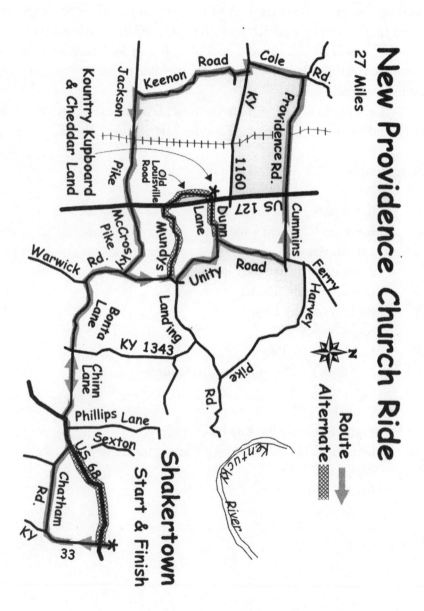

17

New Providence Church Ride

> *Twenty-seven or 29 miles. At least one significant hill. Some traffic on a short stretch of U.S. 68, and crossing U.S. 27. Start at Shaker Village at Pleasant Hill, 23 miles south of Lexington on U.S. 68, or 40 miles south of Frankfort on U.S. 127 and U.S. 68 (with a left turn at Harrodsburg.)*

Another way to get in a good ride out of Shaker Village is to head west toward the country north of Harrodsburg, which includes a couple of very large and elegant farms, and an old Presbyterian church that dates to pioneer days. Also, if you want to take a slight detour, there is a great Mennonite store, where you can get a good sandwich, or buy a lot of good food in bulk.

Not too long ago, it was possible to go out of the front gate of Shakertown, hang a right on U.S. 68, and proceed on this ride without worrying too much about traffic. Lately there have been a few more cars. It's still ridable, but I'm more comfortable on it at some times of day than at others. The Lung Association's Trek now goes down KY 33 to Chatham Lane, and across, to avoid as much of U.S. 68 as it can.

But everything is a trade-off. Chatham Lane—though it is straight on the map, and you can almost count on straight roads to be flat—has a big hill in it. Just when you've hardly had time to warm up. Still and all, I've decided my recommendation is to go that way. It adds about a mile each way to the route. If you're comfortable in traffic, U.S. 68's not a bad way.

Home Farm of Genuine Risk

However you get there, once you've taken a right turn onto Chinn

Lane, you'll start to notice a farm that looks as though it belongs closer to Keeneland. It's **Shawnee Farm**, owned by steel magnate **G. Watts Humphrey**, a mover and shaker in the Thoroughbred racing world.

Humphrey is a director of both the **Keeneland Association** and **Churchill Downs**, and of the **National Thoroughbred Racing Association.** He is vice president, treasurer and director of **Breeder's Cup, Ltd.**, and chairman of **Blood-Horse, Inc.**, publisher of a leading racing periodical.

Humphrey deals mostly in fillies and mares, and he has a reputation as a shrewd buyer, always seeming to spot quality horses before their price has been bid up. His wife owned and bred **Virtuous**, dam of **Genuine Risk**, winner of the 1980 Kentucky Derby, and only the second filly to win that race.

Shrewd or not, somebody must have been asleep at the switch to let **Donna Firestone** get away with Genuine Risk at a yearling sale in 1978, for $32,000. The horse nearly won the Triple Crown. She did win $646,587 in three years of racing. Which is not a bad return on the investment.

Anderson Circle Farm

When you pass KY 1343 on Chinn Lane—or Bonta Lane, as some of my maps call it after 1343—you enter the wondrous domain of Anderson Circle Farm. It's on both sides of the road there, and on one side or another for a pretty good part of this ride.

The farm is remarkable for a number of reasons. For one, it's made up of 30 or so farms—so far—put together over a period of years by a man—**Ralph Anderson**—who grew up on a seven-acre farm in Mercer County. He went off to World War II, was a flight engineer on B-29s, and later went to engineering school at the University of Kentucky.

After working for **General Motors, General Electric**, and other companies, he built a Cincinnati-based engineering services company called **Belcan Corporation**, and apparently got fairly rich.

A second reason the farm is remarkable is that Anderson also is a dedicated history buff and preservationist, and he has restored some great houses and barns on his farm, not to mention fostering archaeological digs and generally making a great contribution to knowledge of Mercer County and Kentucky history.

156

Outdoing the Shakers

So far, he has put together 4,600 acres, a bit more than the Shakers are thought to have owned at their Pleasant Hill peak. He has hired professional managers to make Anderson Circle farm a profit-making operation, and has won recognition for achievement in breeding and crops, just as his Shaker neighbors did before him.

On your right not long after you pull alongside the farm—but not visible—is the **Shawnee Springs** area, once frequented by generations of Shawnee hunters, and later the home place of **Col. Hugh McGary**. It was McGary who urged settlers from the area into an obvious ambush in the 1782 **Battle of Blue Licks**, and got 72 of them killed.

Anderson and his wife, **Ruth**, found an old barn of mortise and tenon construction and moved it to the Shawnee Springs site to be preserved as a unique guest house, with no interior painting, and one wall that is largely glass to make the magnificent view ever accessible to his guests.

Also near the springs is the farm's **Schuler Cabin**, which was threatened by destruction down in Metcalf County a few years ago, and purchased by the Andersons to be reassembled here.

Wildwood and Walnut Hall

Some distance off to the left across from Shawnee Springs is **Wildwood**, the second house the Andersons restored. It is High Victorian Italianate, and dates from the 1860s. It serves as a home for the Andersons' farm manager.

Wildwood was the home of a Mercer County character named **Will Goddard**, who seems to have been called "Uncle Will" most of his life. He was an unreconstructed rebel, and was jailed for a time during the Civil War for aiding and abetting confederates. He hated Yankees for the rest of his life, though he got along well with most other people. He wore white suits with white dusters, and broad-brimmed white felt hats.

Rounding the bend and pedaling on up Warwick Road, you will come to **Walnut Hall**, the Andersons' own home when they are on the farm. It is an 1840s house, Greek Revival in style. When the Andersons bought the farm it is on, it was used to store hay and grain, and chickens

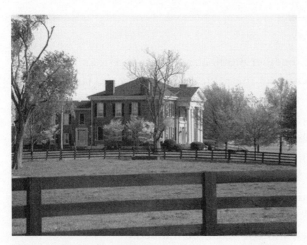

Walnut Hall, the restored 1840's home of Ralph and Ruth Anderson of Anderson Circle Farm.

roosted there.

Doing it Right

The Andersons assembled a team for the restoration, made up of architects from his company, an interior designer, and some very preservation-minded local contractors. It worked out so well he subsequently used the same team for Wild-wood and other projects, and in fact offers their combined expertise in restoration of valuable old buildings for hire to other people.

To get modern heating and plumbing in the place, they installed two complete sets, one in the attic above the second floor and the other in the basement below the first floor, to avoid ductwork that would detract from the period correctness of the restoration.

They buried the wiring by chiseling out groves in the 15-inch thick brick walls, then plastering them over. They scoured the countryside for brick and stone to match the walls and foundation where repairs were needed.

When they scraped all of the layers of paint off the woodwork, they found it was all walnut, and still in good shape. It sounds like a fantastic house. They found a secret stairway from what had been the master bedroom on the first floor to one of four bedrooms on the second floor.

Decision Time

You can get a good look at Walnut Hall through the iron gates at its front, where Warwick Road meets Mundys Landing Road. It is at that juncture that you have to decide if you want to take the side trip over to the Mennonite store.

It is well worth the trip, even though it adds about 2 miles to the route. I made it an alternate because it involves a bit of a tricky crossing of U.S. 127, a very busy road. You will cross it twice on this route anyway, but you have a straight shot across in both cases.

To get to the **Kountry Kupboard**, you have to ride along the highway for a short distance, and then cut left onto Old Louisville Road, which runs almost parallel to 127, up the other side. Be careful. Old Louisville rejoins 127 at the store, but you have a straight shot to get back across there.

The store's hours are 8:30 to 5:30 every day except Wednesday, Saturday and Sunday. It closes half an hour early on Wednesday and Saturday, and is closed on Sunday. The food is great, and there's a public rest room.

The Farm's Front Door

If you do go to the store, Anderson Circle Farm will be on your right the whole way. At the store, if you look back across the highway and up the hill, you'll see a couple of carefully-thought-out and crafted barns, topped by cupolas and joined at one end. That's Anderson Circle Farm's front office, built in the 1990s, with a show and sale barn for the farm's registered Angus cattle.

On to New Providence

If you don't go to the store, you will take a short chunk of Mundys Landing Road across the front of Walnut Hall, and turn left on Unity Road. If you do go to the store, you'll join Unity Road by means of Dunn Lane. In any case Unity will soon bring you to Cummins Ferry Road, which takes you over to U.S. 127, which **New Providence Church** fronts.

The church was founded by a group connected with the **McAfee brothers**, who explored this country and then settled here as contemporaries to Daniel Boone and John Harrod. During a 1773 scouting trip a group of them were near starving on their way back to Virginia, when providence provided them with a deer for **Robert McAfee** to shoot.

They remembered it later after they'd settled here and were forming a church, so they named it New Providence. Their first building went up in 1785, three-fourths of a mile east on Cummings Landing Road. This replacement structure was finished in 1864.

The Grave Yard

Actually, my favorite part of the church is its cemetery, about a mile further after you cross U.S. 127. The road there is called Providence Road. The cemetery is on the left. It includes the graves of eight men who fought in the Revolutionary War, and a lot of other interesting old graves.

The route proceeds west a ways, then turns south on Cole Road, jogs left, then right at KY 1160, and takes Keenon Road down to Jackson Pike. Jackson becomes McCrosky Pike after it crosses U.S. 127 again. And that takes you back to Warwick Road, where you can retrace your steps to Shakertown.

And now you know something about the countryside.

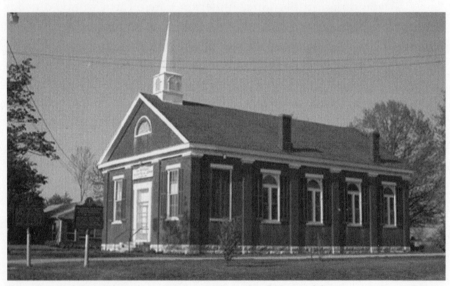

New Providence Church on U.S. 127 north of Harrodsburg.

Route Sheet

0.0	Leave parking lot at Shakertown. Cross U.S. 68 on KY 33.
1.2	Left on Chatham Lane. Hill
2.8	Left on U.S. 68
3.4	Right on Chinn Lane.
4.9	Cross Curry Road (KY 1343).
6.0	Right on Warwick Road
7.7	Right on Mundys Landing Road, past Walnut Hall
7.8	Left on Unity Road
9.0	Right to stay on Unity Road
10.4	Left on Cummins Ferry Road (KY 1933)
11.5	Providence Church. Cross U.S. 127. Be careful.
12.3	New Providence Cemetery on left
13.6	Left on Cole Road. Hill
14.6	Left on KY 1160
14.7	Right on Keenon Road
17.0	Left on Jackson Pike
19.0	Cross U.S. 127. Be careful. Becomes McCrosky Pike
20.3	Right on Warwick Road
21.1	Left on Bonta Lane
23.5	Left on U.S. 68. Be careful.
24.1	Right on Chatham Lane. Hill
25.7	Left on KY 33
26.9	Back at start

There are two alternatives. One takes U.S. 68 out of the parking lot, saves a mile, and avoids a big hill on Chatham Lane. But it puts the rider in moderately heavy traffic on U.S. 68 for a longer period.

The second alternate takes Mundys Landing Road to the left at Walnut Hall (at mile 7.7 in the ride), crosses U.S. 127, and takes Old Louisville Road up to Kountry Kupboard store. It crosses U.S. 127 again and returns to the route on Dunns Lane. It is a 3.2-mile loop that adds about 2 miles to the trip.

Harrodsburg-Cornishville Ride

36 Miles

18
Harrodsburg-Cornishville Ride

Thirty-six or 38 miles. A few significant hills. Moderate traffic. Start at Old Fort Harrod State Park in Harrodsburg, 32 miles south of Frankfort on U.S. 127.

This ride combines a taste of the rich history of old Fort Harrod, which really was an equal with Fort Boonesborough in the early advancement of civilization beyond the eastern seaboard, and a long ramble through the delightful Mercer County countryside up toward Anderson County.

It's mostly on the edge of the real Bluegrass horse country, but it shows what else has been done with the rich agricultural land that led pioneers such as John Harrod to risk all in a battle with the Indians and the British to get a toe hold here.

What you'll see on this trip, along with horses, is a lot of goats. **Mercer County Agent Tony Shirley** told me they are mostly of the Boer variety—meat goats rather than dairy animals—which have been a growing source of income as tobacco declines with increased purchases by cigarette companies of foreign burley tobacco.

Shirley said goats are an ideal new crop for areas where tobacco has been grown, because they fit well into the landscape. They don't mind side hills and they graze on bushes and small trees. As with tobacco, even a small farm can make money with goats. The meat is in increasing demand in growing ethnic markets.

Along with the rural countryside, this ride takes you through numerous small towns, some of them with the great old country stores. You will encounter a climb or two—or, as my friend David Runge says, "an

163

altitude adjustment opportunity." Keeps it from being dull.

Start with the Fort

The ride starts on West Broadway in the parking lot for the 1927 replica of Fort Harrod. Though Fort Boonesborough has had more play in the media—starting with a book by **John Filson** in the 18th century and continuing up to television—Fort Harrod was every bit as important in the establishment of Kentucky and the U.S. west of the Appalachian mountains.

John Harrod, who led 31 men to the site in 1774, was Daniel Boone's equal as a woodsman and explorer, and he had been in the country at least as early as Boone. He led his group down the Ohio River in canoes, then 100 miles up the Kentucky River, and across country to the headwaters of the **Salt River**.

They laid out a town and built cabins in 1774, but ultimately had to clear out because of Indian pressure given a boost by **Lord Dunmore's War** back in Virginia. But they returned the next spring, arriving two weeks before Boone reached Boonesborough with his axemen, and established the first permanent settlement west of the mountains. It ultimately become much more of a town than Boonesborough ever was.

Intrepid Pioneers

The pioneers at Harrodsburg fought off their share of Indian attacks, notably in 1777, that "year of the three sevens" when Kentucky civilization hung on by a thread. Harrod was a noted military leader as well as settler, and he participated in a number of retaliatory raids against the Indians beyond the Ohio.

He ultimately became a prosperous landowner, which was always Daniel Boone's goal, before he disappeared on a hunting trip—in search of the legendary Swift's silver mine, by some accounts—in 1792. His body was never found.

Harrodsburg also was the seat of **George Rogers Clark**, when he was named to command Virginia's military forces beyond the mountains. It was in one of the corner blockhouses at Fort Harrod that Clark planned his foray into the Illinois country, which broke British power there and won the Northwest for the U.S.

Harrodsburg also was the home of **William Poague**, an accomplished woodworker who produced all the buckets, churns, milk pails and other wooden equipment the pioneers needed. His wife, **Ann Kennedy Wilson Poague Lindsay McGinty,** also was inventive, teaching pioneer women to spin cloth out of nettle lint and buffalo wool. And she married new husbands as fast as the Indians could kill the old ones.

Jane Coomes taught at the first school west of the mountains, which was built inside the Harrodsburg fort. She used wooden hornbooks, and a mathematics text she had hand copied before crossing the mountains.

The replica fort offers tours from 8 a.m. to 5 p.m. March through October, and 8 a.m. to 4:30 p.m. from the first of November to the middle of March. Admission is $4 for adults and $2 for children over 6. Children under 6 get in free.

Out into the Countryside

West Broadway and West Lane will get you up to Cornishville Road, also called KY 1989. Take that out to Oakland Lane. Notice Mt. Pleasant Road as you pass it on your right. That's a road that lives up to its name, one you should keep in mind for future exploring in this area.

Oakland Lane is in an exurban area—out in the country but mostly residential—and it will take you down to KY 152 and a right turn that will take you through Rose Hill, and give you some options. I'm suggesting a turn on Johnson Road and up to KY 1989 again and Brewers Mill Road.

You can get to the same place by staying on KY 152 a ways farther and turning right up Bruners Chapel Road and taking that to Brewers Mill. They're both lovely roads. The Bruners Chapel route is two miles farther, which is one reason I've made it the alternate.

It often is used by the American Lung Association's Shakertown Trek riders, under the guidance of noted bushwhacker—which is to say, finder of good, remote roads—David Runge. They usually take it the other direction, though, I think.

The roads you are about to traverse, up and around through **Cornishville, Tom, Duncan, Terrapin, Mayo** and **Bohon,** are often touched by the Lung riders, and by another group Runge is associated with. That group—called **Bag Balm** for an ointment known to soothe the chafing of long miles in the saddle—is loosely led by Jim Moyer, a federal magistrate judge in Louisville and also a noted seeker of remote byways by motorcycle and bicycle.

Watch for the Landmarks

The people who ride these roads have discovered a few picturesque items of interest that never seem to change. A short time after you turn off KY 1989 onto Brewers Mill Road, you will see the old **Brewers Mill**, which is one of the reasons I chose this route. A ways farther, after a right turn on Bushtown Road, you pass a hilly farm with a lot of those goats County Agent Shirley spoke of.

After that, there's a rusty old iron tank hanging from a tree by a chain, twisting slowly in the wind. **Donald Litteral**, at the **Trading Post** in Cornishville, told Dave Runge and me that the man who owns the hanging tank got a new tank. He backed up under that tree and hoisted the old one off his truck, and then pulled out to put the new one on. And so far he has just never gotten around to taking the old tank down.

A bit past the tank, on Bushtown Road, there is an overview that gives you a nice view of Cornishville in the valley below. It really looks good, nestled along the **Chaplin River,** a few houses in the trees, a church steeple poking up. Be sure to watch for it.

You Meet Interesting People

Once when Runge and I rode down the hill into Cornishville, there was a shirtless man standing on a sort of concrete platform near the river, a place where a building had been. He had a 1.75 liter bottle of vodka in one hand, and a jug of Gatorade in the other. He appeared to be inebriated.

He demanded that we come over where he was. Said he wanted to ask us something. There were two of us, so we went. "Why do you ride those damn things?" he asked. It was as if it was just something he'd always wondered about.

I told him bikes are a really good way to see the countryside. For example, I said, Cornishville really looks good from up there on the ridge.

He looked incredulous. He said he guessed you don't notice that sort of thing when you live in a place.

Runge, never one to let an opportunity pass, offered that "You meet interesting people," when you ride. I think I flinched, but if the man had any idea that we might be accusing him of being "interesting," it didn't show on his face.

You Can't Be Too Careful

We talked some more, and I asked him a question. "How can you drink that stuff straight?" I actually meant the Gatorade, which a lot of cyclists dilute with water to cut the chemical taste.

"You gotta replace them ultralites," he said, once he understood the question. He meant electrolytes, of course, those trace elements that become depleted when a person sweats a lot. You do have to replace them, and you can do it with Gatorade, or with beer. So I still think he was doing it wrong.

The Trading Post at Cornishville, incidentally, has sandwiches, cold drinks, snacks and fresh fruit, but no public rest room. It's open from 7 a.m. to 8 p.m.

Grapevine Church

There is nothing left at the village of Tom any more except the **Grapevine Christian Church**, nestled along the bank of the Chaplin. It is a charming church with an ancient cemetery that really deserves a little time.

After that, prepare to climb a bit.

Soon you'll come to Duncan, Ky., and **Wallings Grocery, Hardware and Feed Store**. Runge swears by sandwiches made there by Barbara. There also are soft drinks and snacks. It's open from 6:30 a.m. to 8 p.m. Monday through Saturday, and from 1 to 6 on Sunday. But it doesn't have a public rest room.

There's a steep, winding downhill less than a mile out of Duncan on the Fairview Road. Be careful.

U.S.S. Minnow

A mile or so past the downhill, there's an old bicycle in the bushes on your right. Some years ago, somebody leaned his bike against the fence there, and never went back for it. The vines took over both the fence and the bicycle, so now it's a sort of sculpture. See if you can spot it.

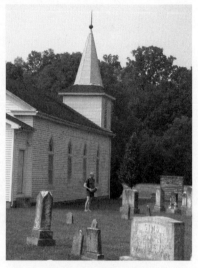

A bit past that is the wreck of an old boat that will never navigate again. Runge has tried to persuade a succession of Trek groups that it is the **U.S.S. Minnow**, the boat that left **Gilligan** and friends stranded. I don't think he's had much success. The views along the road through this stretch are very nice.

There's another grocery in Mayo, and some very nice riding down KY 1160, Hopewell Road, and KY 390. Cornishville Road, West Lane and West Broadway will get you back to the fort.

Dave McGinty examining stones in the cemetery of Grapevine Church at Tom, Ky.

Route Sheet

0.0	Left on Broadway from Fort Harrod parking lot
0.4	Right on West Lane
0.8	Left on Cornishville Street (KY 1989)
1.0	Left to stay on 1989
3.5	Left on Oakland Lane
5.7	Right on KY 152
6.9	Right on Johnson Road
10.8	Left on KY 1989
11.0	Left on Brewer's Mill Road
11.5	Old mill
12.4	Big hill

13.0	Straight on Huffman (Brewers Mill turns left)
13.3	Tank hanging from tree
13.9	Bear right on Bushtown Road.
14.2	Bear left to stay on Bushtown. (Watch for Cornishville overview on the right).
14.6	Cornishville. Jog right, then left on KY 1941.
18.5	Grapevine Church at Tom, Ky.
18.6	Big hill
19.2	Cross KY 390 at Duncan. Wallings Grocery. Continue on Fairview Road.
22.3	Right on KY 1160
24.3	Terrapin. Right to stay on KY 1160
25.5	Mayo
27.2	Right on Bohon Road
28.1	Left to stay on Bohon. Parsons Lane is right.
29.3	Cross Jackson Pike.
30.5	Bohon. Left on KY 390
34.5	Right on Moberly Road (KY 390)
34.7	Left on Cornishville Street (KY 1989)
34.9	Right on West Lane
35.4	Left on Broadway
35.9	Back at start

Alternate passes Johnson Road at mile 6.9 to continue on KY 152, right turn on Bruners Chapel Road at 7.9, to Bushtown at 11.9, then right on Brewers Mill Road, to join the main route with a left onto Huffman Road at 12.5 miles. It adds two miles to the trip. So you can keep track of milage beyond the intersection of Brewers Mill and Huffman by adding 2 miles to each point on the route sheet.

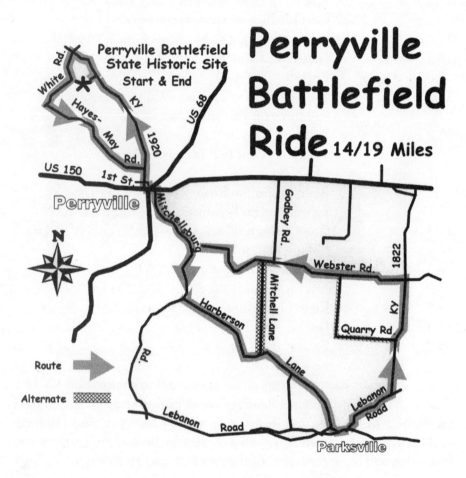

Perryville Battlefield Ride 14/19 Miles

19

Perryville Battlefield Ride

Fourteen or 19 miles. Little traffic and few hills. Start at Perryville Battlefield State Historic Site, two miles out of Perryville on KY 1920. Perryville is 44 miles southwest of Frankfort, on U.S. 127 and U.S. 68, with a right turn at Harrodsburg.

The countryside in and around the little **Boyle County** town of **Perryville** is such a good place to ride a bicycle that it's hard to believe it was a scene of incredible noise, confusion, chagrin and agony in the summer of 1862.

But the battle fought here between the blue and the gray was not only the most significant Civil War engagement in Kentucky. It might well have determined the outcome of that war. So it's interesting to think about from this distance in time.

You could have a perfectly good ride of about 10 miles by just riding out around the battlefield and then down into the town, and pedaling around to look at the historic signs and old buildings.

But just in case you want a little more of a ride, Dave Runge and I scouted out a few more roads to put together a ride that's about 20 miles, or 14 if you take the short cut.

Or, if you really want to get some miles in, you could keep going past White Road on KY 1920, which is also called Mackville Road, and then take Fallis Run Road, New Dixville Road (KY 1941) and Rose Hill Lane, up to the route of the Harrodsburg-Cornishville Ride on KY 152. It's 11.5 miles up to the route, and the route itself is 35 miles. See the last chapter in the book for connections between any ride in the book, and any other ride.

But First, Here's Why They Did It

The Civil War was not going well for the Confederacy in this part of the country in the summer of 1862. Union forces had driven the rebels out of Kentucky, and had all but driven them out of Tennessee, land they couldn't afford to lose. **Federal General Don Carlos Buell** was down in **Middle Tennesee** with 50,000 men threatening to finish the job there.

The Confederates developed a plan to invade Kentucky, which they thought would force Buell out of Tennessee. The Confederates also thought—with considerable encouragement from the Bluegrass's John Hunt Morgan, among others—that they would win the hearts and minds of the Kentucky countryside as well, recruit a lot of new soldiers, and get some new horses.

With Kentucky and its resources on the Confederate side, they thought Lincoln would have to sue for peace, and the war would end. So **Confederate Major General Edmund Kirby-Smith** entered Kentucky from Knoxville, knocked out a Union force at Richmond, and took both Lexington and Frankfort. The rebels installed a Confederate governor, **Richard Hawes**, in Frankfort to give sympathetic Kentuckians somebody to rally to.

Meanwhile, **Confederate General Braxton Bragg** led 32,000 Southern soldiers from **Chattanooga** up through **Bowling Green** and captured a federal garrison of 3,000 men at **Mundfordville**, which is a good chunk of the way toward **Louisville**. Sure enough, Buell headed back for Kentucky with his army.

Uh Oh.

But Buell kept on going, all the way to Louisville—with Bragg moving over to Bardstown to get out of the way—and he picked up another 28,000 men. Then he turned and headed back for the Confederates. He sent 20,000 out the Shelbyville Road to deal with Kirby-Smith at Frankfort, and took 58,000 after Bragg at Bardstown.

Bragg had gone over to Frankfort for the installation of Hawes and to confer with Kirby-Smith, and his soldiers fell back before Buell's advance on Bardstown. Bragg ordered both Confederate armies to concentrate north of Harrodsburg, where he expected to do battle. But Confederate troops got tangled with Federals near Perryville as both sought out the same source of water. It was early October.

Bragg thought most of the federal force was headed for Frankfort, and he didn't know how big an army he faced at Perryville. He ordered an attack. His Confederates fought well, and won ground. But after the fighting stopped at dusk, the peril of their situation became more clear. Bragg and his troops backed away during the night, and ultimately left the state. The South's Kentucky strategy had failed.

Bivouac of the Dead

Meanwhile, back on the battlefield near Perryville, a full moon showed the carnage of the day's fighting—510 Confederate dead, and 845 Union dead. Thousands of wounded on both sides moaned and shrieked on the bloody ground. Witnesses said it was a sight nobody should ever see.

"Bodies of the men and horses lay scattered about the fields, and by the roadside, every house and barn was filled with maimed and dying and the dead. Many of them were in the most horrible condition that the mind can conceive. Some were shot through the head, body or limbs, others mangled by fragments of shell and all suffering the greatest torments," wrote a soldier whose name has been lost.

The Union army buried its dead and moved on, leaving the Confederates on the field. It was up to farmer **Henry P. Bottom**, in whose pastures the armies had fought, to organize a group of slaves and civilians to bury the Confederates. He was much honored for it in the south, and no doubt deserved it. But there was little else he could do. How does one farm around hundreds of unburied bodies?

Head Out Mackville Road

The ride route goes left out of the entrance to the park—which has a gift shop and public rest rooms—and up Mackville Road to a left on

White Road. You are essentially circling the battlefield, and there are all kinds of explanatory markers along the way to explain to you what happened in different parts of the battle.

You'll be struck by the green, green grass, the old buildings, and the beauty of the countryside. The route takes you down into Perryville, a charming town. I loved the house at the corner of First and Buell streets, with its gingerbread, stone chimney, metal roof, and picket fence with flowers all around.

There's a lot to enjoy on both sides of the Chaplin River in downtown Perryville. **Merchants Row,** Perryville's antebellum commercial district, is right across U.S. 150 on the west side of the river. Streets on that side were named after the battle for Federal officers, while streets on the east side were named for Confederates.

You can get a bite of something good to eat at **Battlefield Marathon**, just a bit up 150. It's open from 5:30 a.m. to 9:15 p.m. daily, except Sunday, when hours are 6 to 8:45.

You can get full meals there, and the broccoli casserole comes recommended. The meatloaf and salmon patties are good, too. There's a public rest room.

On to Parksville

If you head out Bragg Avenue then, you'll soon find yourself in more pretty countryside as it becomes Mitchellsburg Road, or KY 1856. Take a left at Harberson Lane and again on KY 34, to **Sinkhorn's Grocery** in **Parksville**. (Or, if you want a ride about five miles shorter, you can take a left on Mitchell Lane, and then on Webster Road, to head back). You can get a good sandwich at Sinkhorn's—or a soft drink or snack. And you'll meet **Edie Sinkhorn**, the proprietress, who has been a favorite with riders on the American Lung Association's Shakertown Trek, which comes through here every September. There's a public rest room.

The way back by Lebanon and Webster Roads offers a couple of opportunities for looping around and alternating legs. It's all nice country. Eventually, you head back up through Perryville and out Jackson Street, or KY 1920, and back to the battlefield parking lot.

Route Sheet

0.0	Leave the Battlefield parking lot.
0.3	Left on KY 1920
0.8	Left on White Road
1.9	Left on Hayes-May Road
3.6	Right on Jackson Street (KY 1920)
4.2	Left on West First Street
4.3	Right on N. Buell Street (which is not signed at that intersection)
4.4	Left on U.S. 50
4.5	Right on Bragg Avenue (KY 1856)
6.5	Left on Harberson Lane
7.5	Pass Mitchell Lane on left.
8.7	Left on KY 34. Sinkhorn's Grocery
8.8	Bear left to stay on KY 34. Some traffic. Be careful.
9.9	Left on KY 1822
10.7	Pass Quarry Road on left.
11.7	Left on Webster Road
12.1	Nice old one-lane bridge
13.8	Left to stay on Webster. Straight is Godbey Road
15.4	Right on KY 1856
16.2	Left on U.S. 50. Battlefield Marathon store.
16.3	Right on N. Buell
16.4	Left on W. First
16.5	Right on Jackson Street (KY 1920)
18.2	Left into park
18.5	Back at start

(Short cut at Mitchell saves 5.1 Miles)

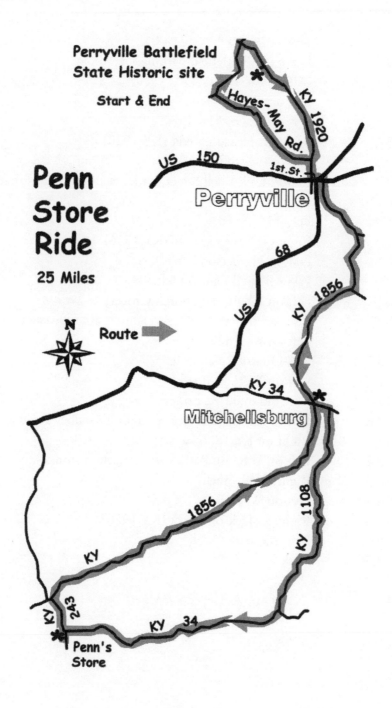

Perryville Battlefield
State Historic site

Start & End

Hayes-May Rd.

KY 1920

US 150

1st. St.

Perryville

Penn
Store
Ride

25 Miles

68

KY 1856

US

N

Route ➡

KY 34

Mitchellsburg

1856

KY 1108

KY

KY 243

KY 34

Penn's
Store

20

Penn Store Ride

> *Twenty-four miles. Two significant hills, and tricky downhills. Light traffic. Start at Perryville Battlefield State Historic Site, two miles out of Perryville on KY 1920. Perryville is 44 miles southwest of Frankfort, on U.S. 127 and U.S. 68, with a right turn at Harrodsburg.*

Penn's Store, which is just inside **Casey County** at the Boyle County line, not far from **Gravel Switch**, is a dilapidated old country place that is famous for being famous. But it's still real.

Arts and crafts and Penn's Store t-shirts have mostly replaced the canned goods, and flour sacks and men's, women's, and children's shoes that used to line the shelves and sit on the warped old floor. But the old batten boards still keep the wind out, and the tin roof is good against rain.

And the old Warm Morning Model 521 stove still burns wood and coal when the place needs heating, and people still warm themselves around it, and swap stories. The cash register is still a cigar box. **Jean Penn Lane**, a direct descendant of **Gabriel "Jack" Penn**, who bought the store in 1850, still sits behind the rustic old counter.

According to magazines such as *Kentucky Living, Southern Living, Country America,* and *Playboy,* which all have written about the store, that makes it the oldest country store in America run by the same family.

The Outhouse

It was probably the outhouse that drew Playboy's attention to the store. For the first 150 years or so, Penn's had no rest room for customers.

But it was starting to get visitors from considerable distances, drawn to the growing fame of its rusticity, and in 1992 then-owner **Haskell "Hack" Penn** judged it was time.

In fact, **The Tarter Gate Company**, in **Dunnville, Ky.**, almost all the way across the county, donated poplar lumber for the project, and two Dunnville men—**Bill Trammell** and **David Tarter**—designed and built the structure. And it is solid, and functional.

Jean Penn Lane, who is Hack Penn's great-niece, had just returned from **Nashville, Tenn.**, where she spent a few years as a songwriter. She thought of asking her friend—songwriter, playwright, and author **Billy Edd Wheeler**—to come to an official dedication. He wrote "Ode to the Little Brown Shack Out Back," which got airtime as a sort of protest song a few years ago.

Chet Atkins

Wheeler said he'd come, and asked if he could bring his friend, guitarist **Chet Atkins** along. That pretty much blew the thing up. The dedication, October 17, 1992, drew 4,000 people to the flat, grassy place along the **North Rolling Fork of the Salt River** where the store sits. And they had a good time.

The Penns decided to make an annual event of it, and they've had outhouse races on the first Saturday in October ever since. They have bands, and they had a car, truck and motorcycle show one year that drew 3,800. "It really needs to be a two-day event," Jean Penn Lane said.

She said people come from all over. She was astonished, she said, to learn through involvement with the event how many outhouse-related celebrations there are in the country. And how innovative outhouse racing technology can become.

Time Marches On

Unfortunately, despite celebrity, it's getting harder to keep Penn's Store open. Hack Penn died a few years ago and his niece—**Alma "Tincy" Penn Lane**, Jean Penn Lane's mother—took over the store, running it with

Jean's daughter, **Dava Osborn Jones**.

But Dava died unexpectedly, and Alma died in 2001. Now the family is down to Dava's twin, **Dawn Osborn Grass**, who lives in Elizabethtown, and Jean Penn Lane.

Jean has a farm nearby with cattle and tobacco that take up her time. So she operates the store on Mondays, Tuesdays and Fridays, and otherwise by appointment. It's best to call ahead: 859-332-7715 or 859-332-7706.

The Ride, and The Climb(s)

I was scouting rides in the vicinity of the Perryville battlefield when I found out one could reach Penn's Store from there, in a round trip of about 25 miles. It sounded good to me. The countryside is beautiful south of Perryville, and also lovely down along the North Rolling Fork, south of **Mitchellsburg**.

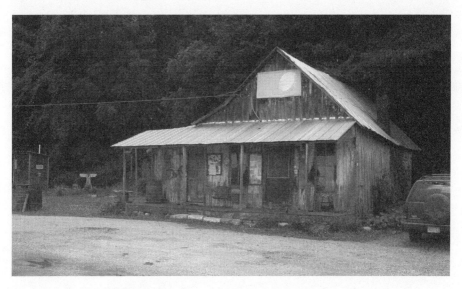

Penn Store, one of Kentucky's famous country stores with its famous outhouse, near Gravel Switch.

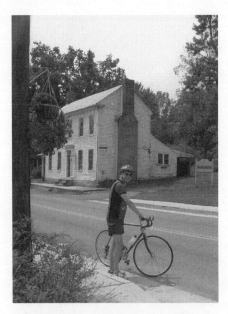

Dave McGinty near an antebellum house in Perryville.

Between Mitchellsburg and the North Rolling Fork, though, is the matter of **Mitchellsburg Knob**, and **Whites Ridge**. Except for those, it's not an overly hilly route. But you run into the knob on KY 1108 just south of Mitchellsburg, and it's moderately steep. Then you go down the other side, which also is moderately steep. And winding. Be careful.

You return to Mitchellsburg via KY 1856. There's a steep hill on that, which I take from the map to be Whites Ridge. Be careful on that descent, too. But once you're down, it's clear sailing back through Mitchellsburg and up KY 1856 to Perryville. There is good food at Battlefield Marathon in Perryville. It's open from 5:30 a.m. to 9:15 p.m. daily, except Sunday, when hours are 6 to 8:45.

There are rest rooms there and at the battlefield. And, Penn's Store, of course, has that famous outhouse.

Route Sheet

0.0	Leave Perry Battlefield State Historic Site, right on 1920.
2.0	Left on First Street in Perryville
2.1	Right on N. Buell Street (unmarked), left on U.S. 150
2.2	Right on KY 1856
6.4	Left on KY 34 in Mitchellsburg
6.7	Right on KY 1108. Start of big hill 1 mile long
7.7	Caution. Steep, winding downhill
10.4	Right on KY 37
11.1	Left on KY 243, cross bridge and right on Penn Store Road
11.3	Store
11.5	Left on KY 243 out of Penn Store Road, and then again
12.2	Right on Ky 1856
16.7	Start of big hill. Only two tenths of a mile, but a little steep. Be careful on the downside.
17.2	Cross KY 34 in Mitchellsburg.
21.4	Left on U.S. 150 in Perryville
21.5	Right on N. Buell and left on W. First St.
21.6	Right on Jackson Street (KY 1920)
21.9	Left on Hayes-May Road
23.4	Right on White Road
24.5	Right on KY 1920
24.8	Back at the park

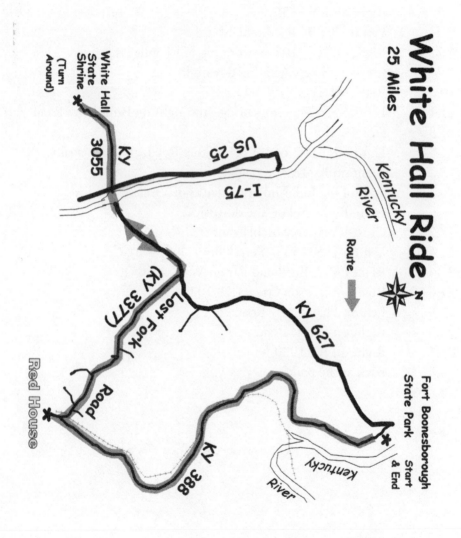

White Hall Ride
25 Miles

21
White Hall Ride

Twenty-five miles. Moderate hills. Some traffic on Lost Fork Road and U.S. 25. Start at Fort Boonesborough State Park, 23 miles southeast of Lexington on I-75 and KY 627.

A lot of the great old antebellum houses that dot the Bluegrass are private residences and not accessible to the public. But there's one storied residence not far from Boonesborough that delivers the flavor of a bygone era, and is open.

It's not just any house. It's the home of **Gen. Green Clay**, a Virginia entrepreneur and contemporary of Daniel Boone who acquired a lot of Bluegrass land and became very rich—operating mills, distilleries, a ferry, taverns, toll roads and warehouses, and growing tobacco and owning slaves. It's the childhood home of **Brutus Junius Clay**, who was a U.S. Congressman, a Kentucky legislator, and a mover and shaker in 19th century Bourbon County, a man who was vigorously both pro-slavery and pro-union.

It was the home of **Laura Clay**, a prominent crusader for women's rights in the late 19th and early 20th centuries.

But most famously, it was the home of **Cassius Marcellus Clay**, emancipationist, ambassador, Lincoln confidant and noted scrapper. While he was a student at Yale University in the 1830s, he heard a speech by **William Lloyd Garrison** that set him on a lifelong course against many of his friends and neighbors on the issue of slavery.

No Shrinking Violet

Clay favored emancipation, the gradual freeing of slaves by legal means, and he freed his own—including, according to one report I found, the great-great grandfather of his prizefighter namesake, who changed his name to Muhammad Ali.

The Richmond Clay spent a good deal of time stumping for his cause, speaking everywhere, heckling pro-slavery speakers at public gatherings, and generally annoying defenders of the South's peculiar institution. He regularly got into knife and gun fights over the issue.

He published a newspaper, *The True American*, in Lexington, for a time, but it drew so much abhorrence that he had to install iron doors, a lot of rifles, and a cannon in his building. Still, a posse of pro-slavery people got into his shop when he was down with typhoid fever, and shipped his press to **Cincinnati**. He continued publishing from there for a time.

A Lincoln Confidant

Clay was himself considered a candidate for president in 1860, but he supported Lincoln, who made him ambassador to Russia. He helped keep Europeans out of the Civil War through his influence in Russia.

During a hiatus in his Russian service, he surveyed public opinion in Kentucky and gave Lincoln assurance that the **Emancipation Proclamation** would not drive the state from the union. He is credited with paving the way for the U.S. purchase of **Alaska**.

Women in His Life

Clay had a stormy marriage with his wife, **Mary Jane Warfield Clay**, who like Clay was a Bluegrass aristocrat. The marriage produced 10 children. But Clay was occasionally linked with other women, including a Russian ballerina with whom he had an illegitimate child.

Clay and Mary Jane separated late in life and divorced when Clay was in his 80s. Clay then married a 15-year-old White Hall servant, **Dora Richardson**, scandalizing proper people in the community.

Officials in Richmond did send a group of men out to White Hall at one point to "rescue" the girl, without success. There is a letter at the house that purports to be a communication from the leader of the posse to the Madison County Judge. It came from **William Townsend's** Clay biography, *Lion of Whitehall*, but curators at the house say they've never been able to authenticate it, and have some doubts about it.

But it is hilarious:

Reporting to the Judge

Dear Judge:

I am reporting about the posse like you said I had to. Judge we went out to White Hall but didn't do no good. It was a mistake to go out there with only 7 men. Judge, the old General was awful mad. He got to cussin and shootin and we had to shoot back, the old General sure did object to being arrested. Don't let nobody tell you he didn't. We had to shoot. I thought we hit him 2 or 3 times, but don't guess we did. He didn't act like it.

We come out right good considerin. I'm having some misery from two splinters of wood in my side. Dick Collier was hurt a little when his shirt-tail and britches was shot off by a piece of horse shoe and nails that came out of that old cannon. Have you see Jack? He wrenched his neck and shoulder when his horse throwed him as we were getting away.

Judge I think you will have to go to Frankfort and see Gov. Brown. If he would send Capt. Longmire up here with 2 light fielders he could divide his men—send some with the cannon around to the front of the house not too close, and the others around through the Cornfield and up around the cabins and spring house to the back porch. I think that might do it.

Fiery to the End

Dora did leave Clay after a couple of years of marriage. She had three more husbands, and died at 34.

Clay continued at Whitehall, defending his castle. When he was

89, three men broke into the place, and Clay met them with his bowie knife and a pistol. He killed two, and one got away.

He died in 1903, in the same bed where he'd been born in 1810. There was a raging storm that night, and a bolt of lightning knocked the head and shoulders off a statue of Henry Clay atop the Clay monument in **Lexington Cemetery.**

The House

White Hall is now a state historic site, open to the public from April 1 to Oct. 31. Hours are 9 a.m. to 5 p.m. every day, except after Labor

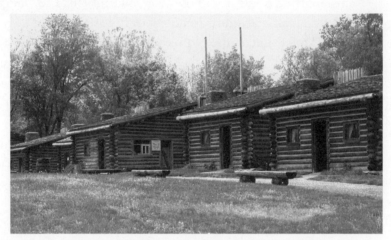

Inside the replica stockade at Boonesborough State Park.

Day, when it's closed Mondays and Tuesdays. Admission is $5 for adults and $2.50 for children. Costumed guides lead the tours.

The house has two parts, a Georgian-style old section built in 1798-99 by Green Clay, and an 1860s section that is an interesting combination of Georgian and Italianate architecture. Mary Jane Clay supervised construction of the latter while Clay was in Russia.

White Hall has a forerunner of central heating systems, with two fireboxes in the basement from which heat is ducted to fireplaces in several rooms. Unlike most houses of its time, it had a bathroom, including a bathtub made of a hollowed-out poplar log lined with copper. Rainwater from the roof was collected in a tank and piped to the bathroom.

Start at Boonesborough State Park

The ride starts at the parking lot at Boonesborough park, over by the swimming pool. Take Ky 388 out to **Red House**, and take a right across the tracks onto Lost Fork Road. That goes over to KY 627, which crosses I-75 and U.S. 25, becomes KY 3055, and goes on out to White Hall.

From there, turn around and go back.

There is a large service station-grocery store at the corner of KY 3055 that has snacks and other foods, as well as soft drinks and a public rest room.

It's all very pretty country. Traffic gets a bit busy on Lost Fork and on KY 627, but the Bluegrass club rides both frequently. Be careful.

Route Sheet

0.0	Leave Fort Boonesborough State Park parking lot, left on KY 388.
6.4	Right on Lost Fork Road at Red House
9.2	Left on KY 627
10.7	Cross I-75, U.S. 25, stay straight on KY 3055.
12.6	White Hall. Turn around
14.5	Cross U.S. 25, I-75, stay straight on KY 627
16.0	Right on Lost Fork Road
18.8	Left on KY 388
25.2	Back at Ft. Boonesborough State Park

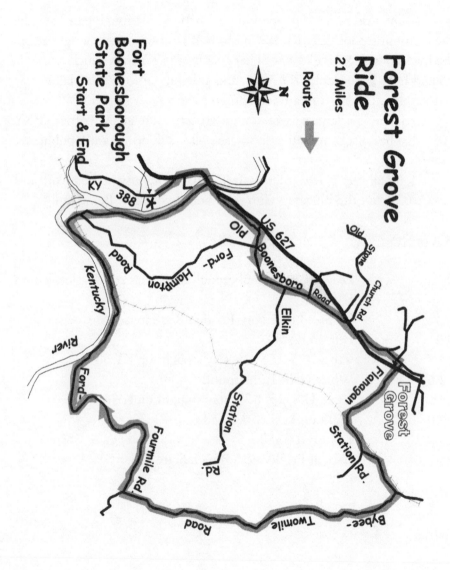

Forest Grove
Ride
21 Miles

Route

N

Fort
Boonesborough
State Park
Start & End

KY 388

US 627

Old Boonesboro Road

Ford-Hampton Road

Kentucky River

Ford-

Fourmile Rd.

Elkin

Station Rd.

Old Store Church Rd.

Flanagan

Forest Grove

Station Rd.

Bybee-

Twomile Road

22

Forest Grove Ride

Twenty Miles. Some hills. Light traffic except for stretches of KY 627. Start at Fort Boonesborough State Park, 23 miles southeast of Lexington on I-75 and KY 627.

This ride takes you easily across the Kentucky River, a feat that could be tough for pioneers. You do have to dodge gravel trucks a bit, so be careful. Start at Fort Boonesborough State Park, take KY 388 out to KY 627, and cross Memorial Bridge.

The shoulder on KY 627 is wide along that stretch, which is a help. And at least the trucks presumably don't mean to menace you. The Indians were flat out out to get Daniel Boone, **Richard Callaway** and others.

If you pause for the historical marker on KY 388 just before you get to KY 627, you will see, in fact, that they did get Callaway, as he was attempting to build Kentucky's first ferry along here in 1780.

Anyway, you'll be crossing the river and riding around in the no man's land across from the old Fort Boonesborough, where the Indians and their English and sometimes French leaders used to gather to attack the fort. Somewhere on this ride you will no doubt cross the trail of the Cherokee chief, **Hanging Maw**, who, with some Cherokee and Shawnee warriors, kidnapped Jemima Boone and **Betsey and Fanny Callaway**, in July, 1776.

But First, Some Background

Daniel Boone first came to this part of the country in 1769, and he explored it extensively, alone and with others, for a couple of years. In March and April, 1775, he came back with 30 axemen, to cut a trail from North Carolina to the mouth of **Otter Creek** on the Kentucky River, for the **Transylvania Company**. That's Otter Creek entering the river just south of the park.

Boone got the men to Boonesborough and got some cabins and a fort started. He lost a couple of men to Indian attacks in the process, but he still went back to North Carolina in the summer for his wife, Rebecca, and his children.

The family had been at Boonesborough almost a year—withstanding occasional Indian mischief—when Jemima and the Callaway girls took the fort's canoe to the river, to soak an injured foot. It was Jemima's. They drifted too close to what is now the Clark County side of the river, and the Indians—who were in the canebrakes there, sizing up the fort—grabbed them and headed for **Shawnee** villages in what is now Ohio.

The Rescue

A group of men from the fort quickly picked up the trail, with some help from the girls, who had managed to drop bits of clothing, sink heels into mud, and break small branches as they passed.

The Indians camped with their captives somewhere around **Winchester**—just north of where this ride goes—the first night. They generally followed the **Warrior's Path**, an old buffalo trace used by Indians for hunting and to travel from Cherokee country to Shawnee country. It went to the Blue Licks and on up to the Ohio River near Maysville.

Boone and the other pursuers caught up with them two days after the kidnapping, and managed a surprise attack on a camp they'd set up to roast a buffalo hump. The girls were unhurt, and the Indians mostly disappeared into the canebrakes.

The Natives Get Restless

About the time the girls were being nabbed, founding fathers were signing the Declaration of Independence back in **Philadelphia**, and the Revolutionary War was growing hotter. For the settlers, that meant serious attacks by Indians stirred up by the British and supplied with ammunition and scalping knives from the royal stores at Detroit.

There were numerous attacks at Boonesborough, Harrodsburg and other nearby stations all through 1777—"the year of the three sevens"—and Boone himself was captured by the Shawnee chief, **Blackfish**, early in 1778 while boiling spring water for salt at Blue Licks.

Blackfish had more than 100 warriors with him when he surprised Boone and some other settlers, and the whole group was headed for Boonesborough. Boone judged that they'd make short work of the fort's defenses.

So, he stalled for time. Boone managed to persuade Blackfish that the fort was too strong, even though the chief's English and French advisors argued that it was an obvious trick. Blackfish decided to wait until later in the year, and to take more warriors. And he adopted Boone as his son, to take advantage of his hunting skills.

Great Siege of '78

Boone bided his time and escaped when he could. He staggered back into Boonesborough in June, to sound the alarm, and to get badly needed repairs made on the fort before Blackfish arrived in September. But Boone had been too convincing. Blackfish brought more than 400 warriors. The fort had 30 riflemen.

There followed considerable negotiation, during which the settlers did a lot of bluffing, and then a lot of shooting. The Indians tried setting the fort on fire, and tunneling under it to blow up a wall. The settlers tried making a cannon out of a log. After 9 or 11 days—accounts vary—the Indians gave up in disgust and went home.

It all happened right near where you are now riding.

Big Hill

Keep all that in mind as you climb the hill on Old Boonesborough Road, which leaves KY 627 a short distance after the bridge. It's not a steep hill, just persistent. But compared to fighting off Indians, it's got to be a piece o' cake.

The old road crosses the new one—KY 627—after a bit, and you have to ride along the busier artery a short distance. Be careful. A short time after that, you reach the store at Forest Grove, where you can reward yourself for the climb.

Janice Brown, the proprietor, offers sandwiches, snacks and soft drinks, in a charming building that dates to 1941. There are no public rest rooms there, but they are available at a Marathon station a couple of miles up the road.

This ride turns right just after the store, though, and re-crosses KY 627, then goes out Flanagan Station Road, and turns right onto Bybee-Twomile Road. It is mighty pretty country—green, rolling fields between the tree lines, tidy Bluegrass farms along the way. Bybee-Twomile climbs a bit, then drops down to Ford-Fourmile Road, giving you a gratifying sense of progress.

Rollin' along the River

Then you ride along Fourmile Creek and the Kentucky River, past a huge generating plant at **Ford, Ky.**—named, presumably for the flat place where settlers crossed the river before there were bridges and ferries. Below this ford, the next place to get across without a boat in those days was at Frankfort.

There are a number of eating and drinking places between Ford and KY 627, most of them catering to fishermen and partiers, and some of them closed down in the winter.

Just before you get to KY 627, KY 418 goes off to the left. That will take you down along the river to the renowned **Hall's on the River Restaurant**, where the specialties are beer cheese and catfish. It's about a mile further on.

Back at the park, you shouldn't overlook the restored fort, a short hike up from the parking lot. Secure your bikes before you go, or roll them up the path. Riding is prohibited.

When it was first opened in 1974, the fort looked Disneyesque. But the logs have grayed since then, and it feels a bit like it might have in 1775

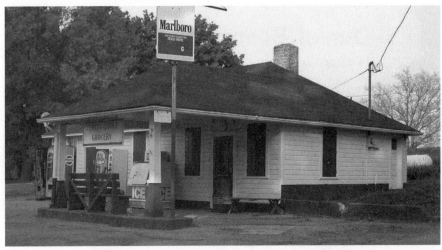

Forest Grove Grocery near Winchester, Kentucky.

in there. Staff in period dress are on hand to tell you about life in the fort. It costs $5 for adults and $3 for children up to 12. Children under six get in free. There's a nice gift shop inside, and public rest rooms.

Route Sheet

0.0	Right from the parking lot at Boonesborough State Park onto KY 388
0.3	Right on KY 627. Be careful. Cross Kentucky River.
1.0	Right on Old Boonesborough Road up the hill
3.8	Right on KY 627 for a short distance. Be careful.
4.0	Left on Old Boonesborough.
4.6	Forest Grove Grocery
4.7	Right on Forest Grove Road. Cross KY 627, and it becomes Flanagan Station Road (KY 1823).
5.7	Bear left in Flanagan.
7.0	Right on Bybee Road, up a couple of hills
12.0	Right on Ford-Fourmile Road
17.5	Pass William C. Dale Power Station in Ford, Ky.
19.5	Left on KY 627 to go back across the river. Be careful.
20.1	Left on KY 388
20.3	Back at parking lot

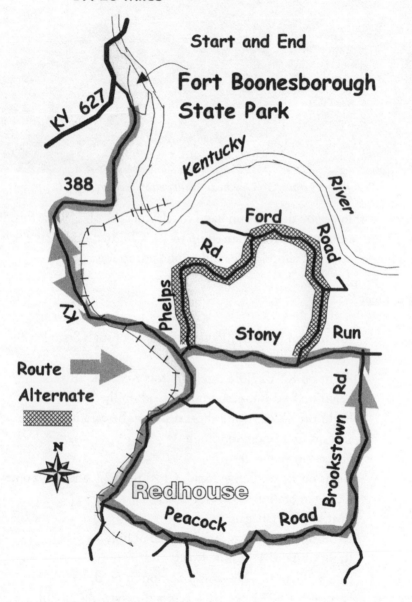

Daniel Boone Ride

17/20 Miles

Start and End

Fort Boonesborough State Park

KY 627

388

Kentucky

River

Road

Ford

Rd.

Phelps

KY

Stony

Run

Route

Alternate

N

Brookstown Rd.

Redhouse

Peacock

Road

23
Daniel Boone Ride

Sixteen or 19 miles. A few hills, depending a little on the route chosen. Light traffic. Start at Fort Boonesborough State Park, 23 miles southeast of Lexington on I-75 and KY 627.

A month or so after *The Courier-Journal* sent me to its **Bluegrass Bureau** in Lexington in 1971, I was tooling around country roads, exploring, and was sort of thunderstruck to see a sign that indicated I was very near Boonesborough. I'd been with the paper a couple of years then and was somewhat familiar with the state's geography, but I hadn't really thought about being near a site of such historic significance.

In north central **Montana** where I grew up, my grandparents were among the first white settlers. History went back about 40 years. Here I was, near the spot where, 200 years earlier, the people who first broke the grip of the eastern seaboard on American settlement had toiled and sweated and fought off redskins.

So I took the old road down into the river bottom, past green pastures and old stone walls, and walked awhile where they walked, read the inscriptions on the monuments, watched the flow of the Kentucky River and raised my eyes to the green hills around.

I'm still in awe of the place.

Red House Hill

A couple of years after that when I had just equipped myself with a bicycle of the proper size, and was trying to learn to use toe clips, I went out for a ride with the Bluegrass bike club that started at Fort Boonesborough State Park.

We started in the big parking lot by the swimming pool, near KY 388, which would be a good place for you to start. The ride went peacefully and pleasantly enough along KY 388 until it got to **Red House,** in Madison County, where it took a turn up Peacock Road.

That was a significant hill for me at the time, and I struggled with the toe clips and the exertion required, and noted with mild dismay that even the women on the ride were sailing blithely past me up the hill. I've learned since on many occasions that pedaling more slowly than some women is nothing to fret about.

But I learned then that some roads are well worth the effort of climbing a hill like that on Peacock Road. Peacock levels out and meanders in a fairly level way along a nice tributary of Otter Creek, then turns left onto Brookstown-Runyan Road, traveling on a sort of bench attained by that Peacock hill.

Then it turns left again, and you come down off the bench on Stony Run Road. I wrote a piece for The Courier-Journal's Sunday magazine about that ride and others I'd discovered in the Bluegrass by then, and this is what I said:

Stony Run Road

Stony Run starts descending gradually back west towards KY 388 and turns into a roller coaster that sails you across old bridges and between stone walls and under canopies of chlorophyll.

A wind with the smell of things growing cools your damp forehead, and you bear down on your feet and ease up off the saddle some and let a little of it blow through there. It's glorious. A cow gives her cud a momentary rest to wonder about you, and you're gone. You glide past old farmsteads and rolling pastures, and nudge the calipers a couple of times to dawdle along a creek bed that picks up the road a ways. It's all silent, except for the creature noises and the whir of your wheels. And you know in your heart that you've worked for it and you deserve it all. You think back to the climb, and to your sniveling misgivings and sexist insecurity, and you feel smug.

Scenic Ford and Phelps Roads

It's also possible to take a right off Stony Run onto Ford Road, and follow it around to Phelps Road and return to Stony Run and KY 388. It's really pretty back in there, and there are some nice ridge-top vistas. But when I rode that stretch for this book, parts of Phelps were so rough I got off and walked. And there was one significant hill back in there. My friend David Runge—for whom the Louisville club has named a certain class of rough though scenic roads "Runge Roads"—loved it.

Taking the Ford-Phelps detour adds about three miles to the route. In any case, you pick up KY 388 again and retrace your steps to the park. Think about what it looked like along here 225 years ago when Daniel Boone first arrived, when the canebrakes had been stomped down by buffalo, and there were more deer than you could shake a stick at.

Route Sheet

0.0	Left out of the parking lot at Fort Boonesborough State Park on KY 388
6.3	Old graveyard on left
6.4	Left on Peacock Pike. Get into a low gear before you turn.
8.3	Bear left along Campbell's Branch.
9.7	Left on Brookstown Road
11.7	Left on Stony Run Road
12.9	Right on KY 388
16.4	Back at the park

The alternate, along Phelps and Ford roads with a right off Stony Run at mile 12.5, adds about 3 miles to the route.

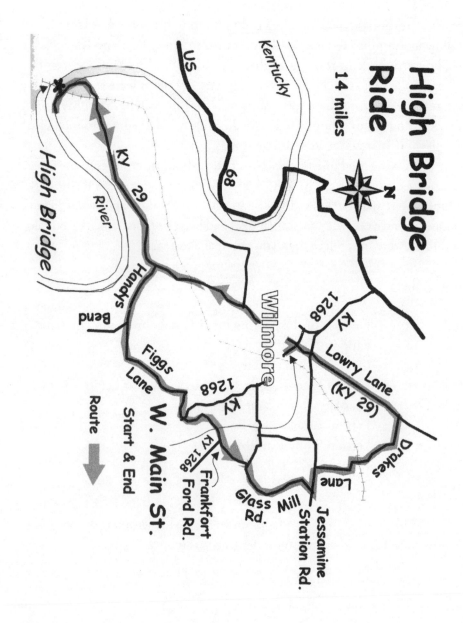

High Bridge Ride
14 miles

24
High Bridge Ride

> *Fourteen Miles. One significant downhill. Moderate traffic. Start on West Main Street in Wilmore, Ky., 16 miles south of Lexington by U.S. 68 and KY 29.*

Several years ago when I was combing through old editions of the Courier-Journal looking for information on the **Wheelmen's Bench**—a 19th century monument near Churchill Downs—I came across this intriguing short, in the Sept. 27, 1897, issue:

"**Miss Mattie Coffman** pedaled across the **High Bridge** and back on the crossties in the presence of a number of people simply for the novelty it afforded."

It was impressive to me, because I knew that High Bridge, which crosses the Kentucky River right in its palisades section, south of Lexington, is really high. When Mattie Coffman did that, it was the highest railroad bridge in the world. Later, I went to see the bridge, and I was even more impressed.

This Mattie Coffman must have had nerves of steel. The bridge has three 375-feet spans, all 275 feet above the water and rocks below. Riding that far on crossties on level ground, without any chance of meeting a hurtling locomotive, would be nerve-wracking enough.

In any case, High Bridge has been a destination for bike rides at least since then, and I'm sure it was long before that. It was built in 1877 for the **Cincinnati Southern Railway**, following a design by **Charles Shaler Smith**.

Twenty years before that, **John Roebling**, designer of the great **Brooklyn Bridge**, had started a span in almost exactly the same place for the **Lexington & Danville Railroad**, which unfortunately became bankrupt in 1857. Roebling's well-crafted stone towers stood beside the Smith bridge until 1929.

Start at Wilmore, home of Asbury College

Wilmore, Ky., is one of those nice little Bluegrass towns, made perhaps even nicer by the godly students of **Asbury College**, a "decidedly Christian"—according to its web page—non-sectarian liberal arts college. The web page says student standards "include abstinence from tobacco, alcohol, illegal drugs and sexual relationships outside marriage." Plus, it says, there's a dress code and a curfew.

The school is highly successful in placing its graduates in jobs or graduate school in broadcasting, music, and journalism fields, and in medical, dentistry and pharmacy schools, among other things.

You can find a place to park on West Main Street near its intersection with Lowry Lane, or KY 29. Then head out 29 toward the bridge, which is almost five miles out.

Taking No Chances

You will notice that the railroad company has gone to great lengths since Mattie Coffman's day to keep people from wandering out on the bridge. There are high, tight fences around the approaches. Graffiti suggests they can be breached, though. But I don't recommend it.

It's awe-inspiring just to stand there and look at the bridge. So many people came to see the bridge in years gone by, some of them detraining from Cincinnati, Lexington, and other points north, that a gathering place grew up there.

It included picnic grounds, a dancing pavilion, a restaurant and riding stables. Cultural and religious meetings there heard from such speakers as **William Jennings Bryan, Billy Sunday** and **Sam Jones**.

The facilities went into heavy decay in the late 1900s, but the dancing pavilion has recently been rebuilt, and new events are being held there under the auspices of the Jessamine County government. To check on events, call the County Judge's office at 859-885-4500.

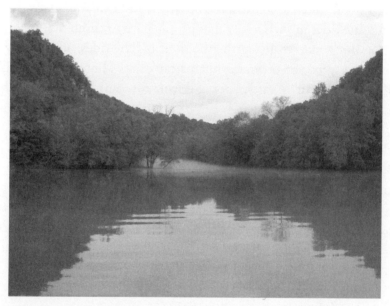

Fog rises on the Dix River, where it flows into the Kentucky under High Bridge.

D. Boone's Tracks

The **Dix River** enters the Kentucky just upstream from the high bridge and you might be able to see its mist-shrouded mouth down through the trees. Daniel Boone had a narrow escape from Indians near there, according to his original biography by John Filson.

The Indians had him trapped against a cliff high over the Dix, and it looked as though they had him. But he looked down and noticed a spindly young tree that looked like it might bend easily. So he jumped off, grabbed the tree by its top, and bent it down to set himself on the ground, where he ran like hell.

Or so he told Filson.

Heading Back

From High Bridge, the route doubles back on itself to Handys Bend Road, where it takes a right and goes over to Figgs Lane. There's a big hill there. Intrepid riders in both the Louisville and Lexington clubs think it's fun to route rides in such a way that people have to climb that hill.

But I may write another book of bicycle rides, and want you to buy it. So I routed you down the hill instead of up. I hope you appreciate it. I also hope you will be careful going down. You can't buy any more books with a broken neck.

Stay straight on Figgs Lane past its first intersection with KY 1268, which would otherwise take you back to downtown Wilmore. About a tenth of a mile past that intersection, the road crosses Jessamine Creek on a picturesque bridge with stone arches.

It is the very bridge chosen years ago for the cover of *Kentucky County Maps*, a book of very detailed maps of every county in Kentucky. It is well-known to bushwhacking cyclists who like to get out into the countryside and find the good stuff.

Food and Drink

Figgs Lane becomes Frankfort Ford Road, which becomes Glass Mill Road. That takes you to Jessamine Station Road, and Drakes Lane, which takes you back to KY 29 and back to the start.

Once there, you have a choice of an assortment of eateries. **Solomon's Porch**, just up Main a bit, is good, and its name is very much in keeping with the biblical flavor of the community. Inside you'll find words of wisdom on the wall. It is a coffee shop and delicatessen, and it smells great.

It's open from 7 a.m. to 9 p.m. Monday through Friday, and from 8 to 2 on Saturday. As is also appropriate in this particular community, it's closed on Sunday. There are public rest rooms.

Further up Main Street, at 319 E. Main, is **Sims Drug Store**, which has a soda shop. You also can get a micro-waved sandwich there. It's open 9 a.m. to 6 p.m., Monday through Saturday. It's closed on Sunday, too. There are public rest rooms.

Route Sheet

0.0	W. Main & KY 29. Go south.
2.0	Pass Handys Bend Road.
4.8	High Bridge
7.6	Right on Handys Bend Road
8.4	Left on Figg Lane (Big downhill. Be careful)
10.1	Pass KY 1268 on left.
10.2	*County Maps* bridge
10.6	Pass KY 1268 on right. Road becomes Frankfort Ford Road.
11.1	Pass Campground Ln. on left. Road becomes Glass Mill Road.
12.4	Left on Jessamine Station Road
12.7	Right on Drakes Lane
14.0	Left on Lowry Lane (KY 29)
14.2	Back at start

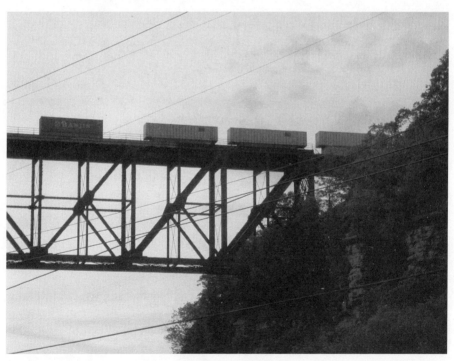

High Bridge, south of Nicholasville, once the highest railroad bridge in the world.

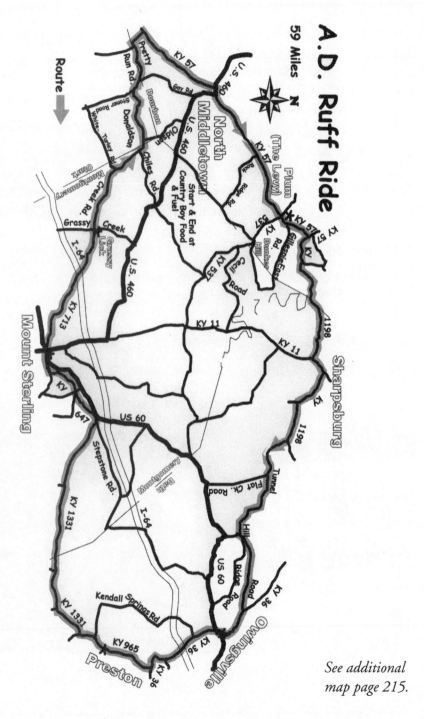

A.D. Ruff Ride

59 Miles

Route

*See additional
map page 215.*

25

A.D. Ruff Ride

Fifty-nine miles. Lots of hills. Moderate traffic, for the most part. Start at Country Boy Food and Fuel Center, North Middletown, Ky., about 26 miles northeast of Lexington. Take U.S. 27 to Paris, U.S. 68 through Paris, and U.S. 460 from Paris to North Middletown.

The Ruff ride is a sort of cyclists' pilgrimage, to the grave of **A.D. Ruff**, a noted Kentucky cyclist of the 19th century. It is the longest and hilliest ride in this book, but the reader is asked to keep in mind that it honors a man who rode his bike from Owingsville to **Yellowstone National Park in 1893**, when he would have been about 66 years old. Now that must have been long and hilly.

Ruff also invented numerous cycling devices, at least one cyclometer and one other invention he patented, according to the research of **Jerry Crouch**, a noted Lexington cyclist. He also was a jeweler and silversmith, and a prominent citizen of Owingsville, and also of Richmond.

Still, I'm thinking that the main reason he is remembered today is that he left $1,000 to the **Kentucky Division of the League of American Wheelmen**, which used it to build a big circular stone bench for cyclists in **Wayside Park** in Louisville, and to erect a distinctive gravestone for him in the Owingsville Cemetery.

Ruff Who?

The stone is an impressive piece of granite, with a slightly-larger-than-life bronze bicycle wheel mounted on it, and the three wings of the old League on the wheel. Years ago, members of the Lexington bicycle club, who are wont to go poking around in old cemeteries, noticed the wheel and wondered about it.

Meanwhile, people also puzzled over the inscription on the wheelmen's bench in Louisville, which still was a popular gathering spot for rides out south from the city when I started cycling with the Louisville club in 1977. There's an inscription on it that says "Erected with the approval of the Board of Park Commissioners by the Kentucky Division of the League of American Wheelmen in Memory of A.D. Ruff." The

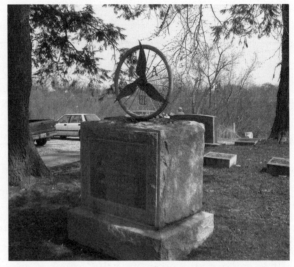

Gravestone in Owingsville Cemetery of A. D. Ruff, a noted 19th century cyclist.

Roman numeral date, 1897, was illegible, and Ruff's name was pretty much so, too.

Nobody could tell me who he was, in any case. I looked through old city directories and library books to no avail. Finally, I went to the **Filson Historical Society** library in Louisville, and found a reference to Ruff in an old bicycling magazine published in Louisville in the 1890s. I wrote a piece about it for the modern league's magazine. Jerry Crouch saw it, remembered the grave, got a date from it, and looked up Ruff's obit. He and I both found more references after that.

I visited the grave early in 2003 with my friend David Runge, and we stopped afterward at **Buster's Diner** in Owingsville for a sandwich. Out of curiosity, I asked our waitress, "Have you ever heard of A.D. Ruff?"

She thought a minute and said, "Didn't they build an arena for him down in Lexington?"

That, of course would be Rupp Arena, named for Adolph Rupp, a noted coach in a whole different sport.

But Not Totally Forgotten

Our conversation was overheard, though, by **Morrow Richards**, an Owingsville banker, who happened to be at the next table. "Did I hear you ask about A.D. Ruff?" he asked. Assured that he had, he said, "Wait here a minute. I want to show you something." He went out to his SUV and came back with a small velvet bag, from which he produced a small silver ladle with the name A.D. Ruff stamped on the back of the handle.

Richards said **Jerome Redford**, a **Georgetown, Kentucky**, silver dealer found it for him, and it's the only surviving Ruff piece either of them knows of.

Start in North Middletown

Not certain how much readers of this book would want to ride a long, hilly way just to see a bronze bicycle wheel, I decided I'd better not start the ride in Lexington, as Bluegrass club riders occasionally do. I checked out a route from Paris, but decided that was long, too, and problematical because of traffic. So I drove out to North Middletown, a small town about 10 miles southeast of Paris on U.S. 460. Paris is 15 miles northeast of Lexington.

I stopped at the Country Boy Food & Fuel Center, which turned out to be pretty much the economic and cultural hub of North Middletown. Timothy Morris, the owner, actually lives in **Mt. Sterling** and drives every Sunday down to Hazard, where he is pastor of a church. He also is a taxidermist, as is clear from various game heads hanging around the store.

His food specialty at the store is a ham sandwich that is very good, and one sees customers leaving his store regularly with whole cases of Ale-8-One, a ginger-flavored soft drink bottled in nearby Winchester. You don't see much of it outside The Bluegrass, but people around here are partial to it. Everybody from the nearby countryside pops in at Morris's store from time to time. You might see **David Dick**—a former CBS correspondent who has written several Kentucky books—there. He lives on nearby **Plum**

Lick Creek.

Morris has a sizable parking lot behind his store, and he said it is okay for cyclists to leave motor vehicles there in order to pedal out into the surrounding countryside. The Country Boy's hours are 6 a.m. to 10 p.m., except Saturday, when they are 7 to 10, and Sunday, when they're 8 to 10.

More Stores

Start the ride by heading up KY 57, which leaves U.S. 460 on the left about a block east of Morris's store. You only get five miles along your journey before you come to the crossroads site of **Plum**, which is also known as **The Levy**, though it's hardly big enough to qualify for one name. **J.D.'s Country Store** is there, and it was proprietor **Wilbur Dale** who told me Plum is also called The Levy. "Don't ask me why," he said.

Janice Dale does the cooking and generally runs the place. Hence, J.D.'s. Besides soft drinks and snacks, the store has an assortment of sandwiches. And there is a public rest room.

You stay on KY 57 for another mile and a half or so, then turn right onto KY 1198. That winds east a ways and runs into KY 11, just south of the town of **Sharpsburg, Ky.** Zip into Sharpsburg and you will encounter **The Sharpsburg Supermarket** on the right—your third store, and you're only 12 miles out. **Sam Habash** sells soft drinks and snacks as well as groceries, and has a public rest room.

He's open 7 a.m. to 10 p.m. six days a week in summer, and 7 to 9 in winter. Sunday hours are 8 to 10 in summer and 8 to 9 in winter.

Out across the Countryside

KY 36 will take a traveler from Sharpsburg to Owingsville, but traffic on it can get a little heavy. For cyclists, KY 1198 is just the ticket. It takes a right a bit past Habash's store, and wends its way east to Tunnel Hill Road— which hooks into KY 36 just north of Owingsville. Expect a few hills along the way.

Take 36 on in to town and take U.S. 60 right and around the corner. It goes into Main Street, which will take you left to Cemetery Road. Just inside the cemetery entrance, you can't miss Ruff's bronze wheel on the left there. There are a lot of other interesting old graves around there, too.

Eat and Talk

You can backtrack a bit then, if you like, and find **Buster's Diner**, for food and conversation. It's open from 6 a.m. to 8 p.m. most days, and on Sundays from 8 a.m. to 6 p.m. "or so." Just around the corner toward the courthouse is **Richardson's IGA**, which has the usual store fare, including sandwiches. Both places have public rest rooms.

It's worth going off the route of KY 36 a block or so to swing around the court house on South Court Street and read the historic signs. **Confederate General John B. Hood** was born in Owingsville. He fought "with distinction" at **Sharpsburg, Fredericksburg, Gettysburg and Chickamauga**, losing a leg at the latter place. He met defeat at **Atlanta**.

Eponymous Colonel

Also on South Court is the former home of **Col. Thomas Deye Owings**, for whom Owingsville is named. He was in the iron smelting business at several places in this part of Kentucky, and was involved in building Ironworks Pike, which hauled iron from around here down to the Kentucky River at Frankfort during the War of 1812. You'll see one of his old iron furnaces south of town, and encounter Ironworks Pike on several other rides in this book.

Owings also organized a regiment for that war, so he was a real Kentucky Colonel. His house was built between 1811 and 1814 by **Benjamin Latrobe**, who also redesigned the interior of the U.S. Capitol after the British burned it in that same war. Henry Clay attended a grand ball here.

One historic marker here says Owings was host to **Louis Philippe of France**. Another says, "Reputedly, in 1814, someone posing as Prince Louis Philippe was a guest here." Keep that in mind when you read historic markers about who slept where.

Pumping Iron

South Court takes you around to the left, back to KY 36, where you'll take a right and head out of town. You go down a hill to cross I-64, and before long you come to the **Bourbon Works**, an old stone smoke stack that was the first blast furnace in Kentucky.

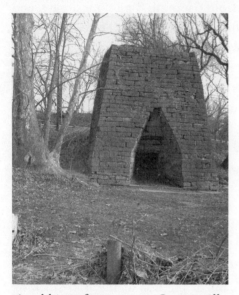

An old iron furnace near Owingsville Ky. It produced munitions for the War of 1812.

It's been standing there since 1791. At first it made utensils and tools for settlers, but war came along soon to boost its profits. It made cannon balls for the **U.S. Navy** in 1810, and shipped iron along the aforementioned Ironworks Pike for use against the British at the **Battle of New Orleans**. Its last blast was in 1838.

While Eastern Kentucky was never **Pittsburgh**, there was a lot of timber for charcoal, native oar, and limestone around here, all of which come in handy for making iron. Kentucky was the number three iron producer in the country in 1830. Eventually the ore and timber ran out, and railroads provided economical transportation of iron from places that could make it more efficiently.

Blevins Store

Take a left off KY 36 onto KY 965 and you'll soon arrive in **Preston, Ky.**, at **Blevins Grocery**, operated by **Helen and Rube Blevins**, who are nice people and moderately famous. The store is known for its loafers, who whittle just to make wood smaller and not to carve anything, through stories in such publications at *The Courier-Journal* in Louisville and public television shows.

You can get cold drinks and sandwiches there, and use the outhouse if you need to. There's a pot bellied stove going if the weather is cool, and there are people sitting around you can talk to.

The week before the third Monday every October, Preston comes alive with a sort of prelude to the Court Day celebration for which nearby Mt. Sterling is famous. A few years ago it was decided that the actual Court Day event had grown too big to do its dog and gun swapping right in Mt. Sterling, so those events were moved to Preston, Helen Blevins said.

Mt. Sterling

Head on down KY 965 to a left on KY 1331, then to such places as **Peeled Oak** and **Howard Mill**. There might be a hill or two in there. Take a left on Stepstone Road and then KY 647 just short of I-64 and U.S. 60, and pedal on in to Mt. Sterling. Take a left on Smith Street and a right on Locust Street to stay off the main drag, then cut right on Queen Street.

Queen Street will take you across U.S. 60, which is Main Street, to a left on High Street, which will take you out of town in the right direction. But look left as you're crossing Main Street, if you're interested in refreshment, or need a break. **Berryman's Pastee Treat**, which is known for its chili and milk shakes, is down there a bit. I'm not sure how that combination will set on your stomach.

Berryman's is decorated in a '50s Coke motif, though, and is a cool place. It's at 305 E. Main. It's open from 6 a.m. to 10 p.m. Sunday through Thursday and 6 to 11 on Friday and Saturday. It has a public rest room.

Adena Mound

Mt. Sterling was named for an Indian mound that was once situated near the corner of Locust and Queen streets, but which is long gone. The town does have another mound though, of the **Adena** culture, which is located just off U.S. 460 at the Bypass—KY 686—about a mile and a tenth off the route I chose for this ride. **Jeff Pratter**, Planning and Zoning Administrator and Building Inspector for Mt. Sterling, assured me that a cyclist could ride that far out 460 without being run over.

I didn't do it, though, because I've seen the mound, and I couldn't find out much about it. It was excavated in the 1930s by **University of Kentucky archaeologist William S. Webb**, who found an intriguing tablet that confirmed the mound as an Adena site.

The Adena flourished in the Middle Woodland period of Kentucky prehistory, from about 500 B.C. to 200 A.D.

They buried important people in mounds and made tablets that you associate at first with something out of **Central America**. But I had a hard time finding out anything else about them, and you won't by visiting the mound, either.

Ubiquitous John Hunt Morgan

Riding your bicycle in this part of Kentucky means you will frequently cross the trail of John Hunt Morgan, a Lexington soldier who raided around Kentucky, Indiana and Ohio and became quite a hero to the Confederacy.

Here in Mt. Sterling, some of Morgan's men robbed the **Farmer's Bank** of $60,000 on the night of June 8, 1864. It was a robbery, and not a burglary, because they went to the home of **J.O. Miller**, cashier, and made him fork over the key to the vault. The money was never recovered.

The bank did sue **Lt. J.F. Witherspoon** after the war, and won a judgment of $59,057.33, leaving us to wonder about the other $942.67. The Court of Appeals ruled, though, that, under the laws of war, robbery was not unlawful, and also, that there was no proof Witherspoon had any more to do with the robbery than other Morgan men.

Anyway, the old Farmer's Bank Building now houses **De De's Gifts**, on Main Street, just a little past Berryman's.

Noted Architecture

Mt. Sterling has some exceptional **Victorian architecture**, and you'll see some of it as you pedal out of town west on High Street. High Street becomes KY 718, once it crosses the bypass west of town, and it will take you back across I-64, to the crossroads community of **Grassy Lick**, about five miles out of town.

You can get a sandwich or a soft drink at the **Grassy Lick Store**, where **Teresa Barnett** is proprietress. You also can get in a card game, or play some pool. But there's no public rest room.

You take a left at the store and then a right almost immediately on Donaldson Road. That's **Grassy Lick Methodist Church** on the corner. Its congregation was formed in 1790, and is the oldest continuous Methodist congregation in Kentucky. Head on out Donaldson Road.

Twists and Turns

It's just good country riding from here. There might be some hills. Take a right on Big Stoner Road about six miles out of Grassy Lick, and stay straight on the aptly-named Pretty Run Road a mile or so later. Then take a right on KY 57 and head back for North Middletown.

You've probably just been on some roads ridden in years gone by A.D. Ruff himself.

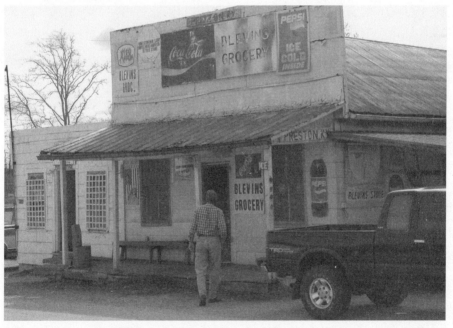

Blevins Store, one of Kentucky's famous country stores, in Preston, near Mt. Sterling, Kentucky.

Route Sheet

0.0	Leave Country Boy Food & Fuel store in North Middleton.
	Left U.S. 460
0.1	Left on KY 57
5.0	Plum (The Levy) Store. Stay on 57
6.4	Right on Ky 1198
10.6	Right on KY 1198
11.5	Left on KY 11
12.0	Sharpsburg Super Market
12.2	Right on KY 1198
13.9	Left on KY 1198
15.1	Stay to right on KY 1198.
15.9	Bear left on KY 1198.
16.8	Bear left on KY 1198.
19.5	Left on Tunnel Hill Rd.
19.6	Keep straight on Tunnel Hill Road.
22.4	Right on KY 36
23.7	Right on U.S. 60 in Owingsville
23.8	Left on U.S. 60. Watch for Buster's and Richardson's IGA.
24.0	Left on Main Street, right on Cemetery Road.
24.1	Ruff grave. Turn around and go back to Main.
24.2	Left on East Main
24.2	Stay straight on Main and then turn left on S. Court. Owings House
24.3	Curve to left and then turn right on KY 36.
25.8	Cross I-64.
26.6	Bourbon Iron Furnace
27.3	Right on KY 965
29.3	Blevins Store at Preston
30.3	Left on KY 1331 (Preston Road)

33.0	Peeled Oak
35.6	Right on KY 1331 at Howard Mill
36.0	Bear left on KY 1331.
38.7	Left on Stepstone Road
39.0	Left on KY 647
40.1	Bear right on KY 647, where Osborne Road comes in from the left.
41.1	Left on Smith Street
41.4	Right on Locust Street
42.0	Right on Queen Street. Pass Main Street and look for stores on left.
42.1	Left on High Street. It becomes KY 713
45.3	Cross I-64.
47.2	Grassy Lick. Left on Grassy Lick Road, then right on Donaldson Creek Road.
53.2	Right on Big Stoner Road
53.6	Stay left. Becomes Pretty Run Road.
54.8	Stay right on Pretty Run.
55.6	Right on KY 57
59.0	Right on KY 460 in North Middletown
59.1	Back at Country Boy

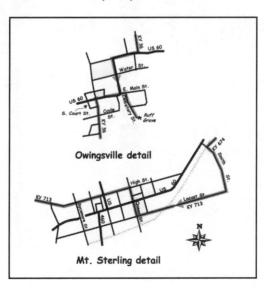

Owingsville detail

Mt. Sterling detail

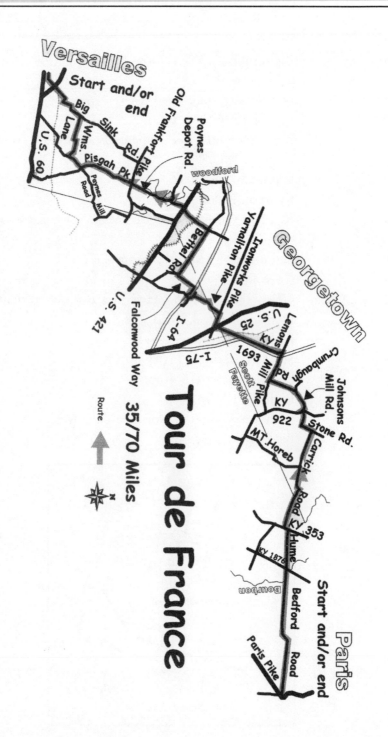

Well, okay. 26
Tour de France

Thirty-five or 70 miles. Moderate hills and traffic. Start at Bourbon County Middle School, which is on the Paris Pike (U.S. 27) on the southwest edge of Paris, 14 miles northeast of Lexington.

In the late 1700s when The Bluegrass was being settled, France was helping Americans win the Revolutionary War, and people were grateful. It was very different from 2003. So French names popped up quite a bit—Paris, Bourbon County, Versailles, etc. The pronunciations might vary a bit, but the honor is clear.

Years later—perhaps in July, but long before any Americans were prominent in the great French classic bicycle race—some club cyclist casting about for a ride, said, "Wait a minute. We could go from Paris to Versailles, and call it the **Tour de France**."

I enjoyed that a lot when I was in the Bluegrass Club in the mid-1970s. And this book was being written in the summer of 2003, when American **Lance Armstrong** was joining four other Tour de France greats by winning his fifth tour—and joining only one other champion by making it five in a row. So I had to put a Tour de France in this book.

Since it follows routes of other rides already in the book, except for a couple of short connectors, I've put it in as a **bonus**. Over the years I think the club's Tour de France has used one route and then another, and I'm not sure this exact route has ever been a club ride. But it gets the job done. Paris to Versailles. Here it is.

A Little Bit of This, and a Little Bit of That

You start with a chunk of the Paris-Beth-Paris ride, throw in a little connector to get past Georgetown and down to a piece of the Equus Run Ride, and then another bit of connector, to pick up a piece of the Big Sink Ride. Then you deviate slightly to ride a chunk of Pisgah Pike that's not on any of the other rides, hook back into Big Sink road, and you're in Versailles.

I've set the mileage to come out right about Huff's Grocery and Deli, which seemed to me to be a good place to meet someone to pick you up. Or, to turn around and go back, if you want to make it a 70-miler. Or you could always do it Versailles-to-Paris.

And there you have it. The Tour de France. Lance Armstrong, eat your heart out.

Route Sheet

Tour de France Route

0.0	Leave Bourbon County Middle School, crossing Paris Pike onto Hume Bedford Road.
5.1	Cross Greenwich Pike.
6.6	Left on Russell Cave Road. Loradale Store.
6.8	Right on Carrick Road
9.6	Cross Mt. Horeb Road.
11.0	Left on Stone Road
12.0	Left on KY 922 (Newtown Pike)
12.3	Right on Johnsons Mill Road
13.2	Stay straight on Crumbaugh Road
14.3	Right on Lemons Mill Road
15.5	Left on KY 1693
18.4	Left on U.S. 25
18.5	Bear right through grocery parking lot to Ironworks Pike.
18.6	Right on Ironworks Pike
19.1	Left on Yarnallton Road
20.2	Jog left, then right to stay on Yarnallton as Hamilton Lane

	comes in on the right. Cross I-64.
20.6	Right on Falconwood Way
21.1	Follow Falconwood around to left.
21.9	Right on Bethel Road
24.1	Left on Paynes Depot Road (U.S. 62)
25.4	Right on U.S. 421, then left to continue on Paynes Depot
26.0	Pass Weisenberger Mill.
26.1	Left to stay on Paynes Depot
27.9	Jog right on Old Frankfort Pike, then left on Pisgah Pike.
30.2	Right on Paynes Mill Road
30.8	Right on Williams Lane
32.6	Left on Big Sink Road
34.5	End at Huff's Deli (or turn around and go back for 70 miles). Or vice versa.

Connections

The rides that make up the Tour de France aren't the only ones in this book that can be combined. You can hook up any of them that are reasonably adjacent. And in my sincere effort to be all things to all people, I'll tell you how.

I've already pulled out some short rides, which I've mentioned previously, for people who are just beginning to ride bikes. There are more such people than there are really experienced cyclists, and I need them to buy this book.

On the other hand, people who ride longer distances are more likely to buy this book just because it's there. So it has to have something for them, too.

As I was gathering information, I talked with **Jack Deacon**, a member of the Bluegrass Cycling Club who does rides like Paris-Brest-Paris, and whose 1982 book, *Cyclin' The Blue Grass*, is one of my prized possessions. He said there's a need for a book of rides that take more than one day to do.

Hook 'Em Up

I didn't think it was in the scope of this book to do many of those. But it occurred to me that, by showing the links between the rides, I could offer routes that can take you from Mt. Olivet to Berea, say, or from Owingsville to Penn's Store, or Switzer to West Irvine.

For that matter, you could make a big loop that would take you from Mt. Olivet to Owingsville, to West Irvine, to Penn's Store, to Switzer, through Paris and back to Mt. Olivet. That would be a pretty long ride.

Here are the main connectors:

Blue Licks Ride to A.D. Ruff and Lonesome Pine Rides
Leave the Blue Licks route at mile 22.9, where Cane Run Road meets Cassidy Creek Road.

0.0   Right on Cassidy Creek Road.

0.9   Right on KY 57

4.3   Left on KY 36

4.4   Right on KY 57

13.5   A.D. Ruff ride goes left on KY 1198. You're at mile 6.4 of that ride.

14.9   Plum, KY.

19.9   North Middletown. Lonesome Pine route goes right on U.S 460 or (to backtrack) stays straight on KY 57. You're at mile 14.5.

Lonesome Pine Ride to Forest Grove Ride
Leave Lonesome Pine route at mile 3.0 in Clintonville and go south on Clintonville Road

0.0   Right on Clintonville Road (KY 1678)

4.1   Jog left on U.S. 60, one-tenth of a mile.

4.2   Right on Venable Road

6.5   Left on KY 1927

7.1   Right on Becknerville Road

9.3   Left on KY 1923

13   Forest Grove. Forest Grove Ride comes in on Old Boonesborough Road, and goes left on Flanagan Station Road. You're at mile 4.7

White Hall Ride to Ferry Ride to Berea
Leave White Hall Ride at KY 627 and U.S. 25. You're at mile 10.7.

0.0	Left (South) on KY 25
1.4	Right on Clay Lane
3.8	Right on KY 1156
8.5	Reach Berea Ferry Ride on KY 169 at Valley View. You're at mile 13.7.

Forest Grove Ride to The Valley Ride
An alternative for getting from the Boonesborough area to the Berea area would be to hook up the Daniel Boone Ride with The Valley Ride, going down the east side of Richmond. I have not had a chance to ride these roads, but riders from the area say they are good. Leave the Daniel Boone Ride with a right onto Hacket Road from Peacock Road just above Red House, which would be at mile 6.5 of the Daniel Boone Ride. Then go:

0.0	Peacock and Hacket
3.1	Left on KY 1986
5.0	Right on Dunbar
5.7	Left on Fourmile Road
5.9	Right on Moberly Number 2 Road
7.1	Jog left on Concord Road, then
7.2	Right on Airport Road.
7.8	Left on Moberly Number 1 Road
9.6	Cross KY 52. Moberly becomes KY 374.
14.4	Reach KY 499, at mile 15.6 of the Valley Ride.

Berea Ferry Ride to Shaker Village and Harrodsburg-Cornishville Rides
This route is all part of the Adventure Cycling's TransAmerica Trail.
Leave Berea Ferry Ride at KY 595 and KY 1295, at mile 30.8

0.0	Right (West) on KY 1295
4.0	Right on KY 1131
4.7	Left to stay on KY 1131
8.7	Left on KY 39
9.7	Right on KY 563
12.8	Left on Jack Turner Branch Road

14.3	Right on KY 1355
21.0	Jog left on U.S. 27. Joe's EZ Foodmart
21.2	Right on KY 1355
21.9	Right on Swope Lane
22.8	Right on Tanyard Road
23.5	Left on KY 753
25.8	Left on KY 152
27.5	Cross Herrington Lake.
32.5	Reach Shaker Village Ride in Burgin at KY 152 and KY 33, at mile 14.2.
37.2	Reach Old Fort Harrod State Park, and the beginning of Harrodsburg-Cornishville Ride.

Old Whiskey Trail Ride to Harrodsburg-Cornishville Ride

Leave the Whiskey Trail Ride where KY 1984 meets Steele Rd, at mile 19.7

0.0	Left (south) on Steele Road
3.1	Right on Milner Road
4.0	Right on U.S. 62
5.9	Cross Kentucky River. Spectacular high railroad bridge on left
8.8	U.S. 62 turns left. Stay straight on KY 44.
9.7	Cross U.S. 127.
11.8	Left on Taylor Road
14.0	Right on U.S. 62
14.7	Left on KY 513
18.8	Right on KY 749
22.5	Left on Cox Road
24.0	Cross Bluegrass Parkway. Cox becomes Bondville Road
24.4	Right on Gash Road
26.0	Right on Kirkwood Road
26.2	Bear left on KY 1987.
26.9	Right on Bardstown Road
29.0	Left on Vanarsdell Road
29.2	Right on Cole Road
32.2	Right on KY1160.
32.7	Reach Bohon Road, hook up with Harrodsburg-Cornishville